Coach, Run, Win

Praise and Testimonials for
Coach, Run, Win

I have had the privilege of knowing Ken Sayles since I first started coaching at San Juan Hills High School in 2011. Ken was one of the coaches I approached for advice since I was new to our league and conference. We met over coffee, and he openly shared at that time that he was still figuring out how to successfully work with the girls. *Obviously,* he figured it out since shortly thereafter, his girls' teams seemed to be winning everything. Now, years later, I learn that that was about the time he started to diligently utilize the Jack Daniels Running Formula with his teams. His book about that journey is an easy-to-read, step-by-step pathway to success and puts into practical terms the Jack Daniels Program—showing any coach just how to achieve the best results with distance runners. I intend to use Ken's book with my own teams. I like the shorter chapters that clearly spell out what to do at each step along the way. Ken Sayles book is the Jack Daniels Running Formula in action!

—**BOB PRICE**, head coach girls' cross-country team at San Juan Hills High, alternate to the 1968 Olympic Team in the Steeplechase and a participant in the Jack Daniels Testing Program

I have read many books on coaching high school cross country in my thirteen-year career coaching high school girls' cross country in south Orange County; some I have valued, while others not so much. Along the way, I always thought I was a detailed head coach, taking pride in always crossing my *t*s and dotting my *i*s. That was, until I read Ken Sayles's book on anything and everything coaching high school cross country, mainly focusing on girls. From training to nutrition, and race prep to all of the numerous nuances coaching this stellar sport, I found his compilation of ideas and knowledge to be informative, thorough, well written, and simple to follow. This is a nuts-and-bolts guide to coaching cross country, focusing not so much on intricate science but rather, the good old day-to-day details of training to dealing with hot days, which many do not think about. I am still involved in this sport—and will be for a while—and I very much want another trip to the State Finals and another Orange County girls' cross-country team title. This book will assist that process. Simply good stuff.

—**DENNIS KELLY**, head coach, girls' cross country and girls' track and field teams at Trabuco Hills High School

Coach Sayles takes a scientific yet practical approach to our sport and is able to translate that to his runners and allow them to understand and believe in the process. His athletes follow his every word, having vested their trust in him, knowing that he truly cares about each and every one of them. In my opinion, Coach Sayles is the epitome of what a high school coach should be: a knowledgeable and experienced teacher, possessing a passion and love for their sport, competitive but humble, a great communicator, a force of positivity, and a rock in the often-tumultuous life of a young person. I have the utmost respect for him as a professional and it has been a privilege to be his colleague and rival—and an honor to be his friend.

—**COACH CHRIS LYNCH**, director of cross country/track and field at Laguna Hills High School, Laguna Hills Cross-Country Invitational

Ken Sayles is a great coach. We have known each other for more than thirty years, and during that time, we always collaborated in the summer months to exchange training plans and ideas and talk about our teams and the upcoming season. He was always willing to exchange his thoughts and materials with me. I was always concerned when we had to race against Capo Valley because I knew they would be ready and well prepared to meet any challenge my team would put up against his teams. His season-long training plans were detailed and well thought-out. His vision was clear and to the point, and he was able to consistently peak his teams when it counted the most at the California State Meet.

—**RICH MEDELLIN**, head coach track and cross country
at Esperanza High School, two-time CIF SS XC
Champions, ten-time CIF SS XC Runner-up
fifteen-time California State Meet finalist

I was Ken Sayles's first high school record holder during his first year as an assistant coach for the Capistrano Valley High School girls' cross-country team. I was immediately impressed with his knowledge of the science of running and his interest in customizing it to each individual runner to maximize their abilities. In the years following my high school career, when he became head coach, he had expanded his knowledge tremendously and created a very successful program with several champions. He has also earned high accolades rewarding not only for his success but also his personal character as a coach. For the 2019 season, I had the honor to start as the new girls' head cross-country coach. I am continuing the legacy of the quality program he has built for over thirty years. Ken has mentored me not only as an athlete over the years, but now as a head coach learning the attributes of how to train athletes to their full potential. I am fascinated with his training philosophies and attention to detail that will continue in our cross-country and distance track programs for many years to come.

—**TRACI MAYNARD**, head coach of Capistrano Valley High School
girls' cross-country and distance track teams

Coach, Run, Win is an excellent guide to all aspects of coaching cross country. As one of Coach Sayles's former athletes, I can personally vouch for the wisdom of this approach to coaching. Specifically, Coach Sayles's data-driven approach to workouts facilitates athletes achieving their full potentials. His administrative structure to running programs places an emphasis on sportsmanship and team building that are equally important to achieving individual and team success.

—**MELISSA BELL**, former Capistrano Valley High School
runner and attorney-at-law

COACH
RUN
WIN

A COMPREHENSIVE GUIDE TO
Coaching High School Cross Country, Running Fast, and Winning Championships

KEN SAYLES
2014 Southern California "Coach of the Year"

NEW YORK

LONDON • NASHVILLE • MELBOURNE • VANCOUVER

Coach, Run, Win

A Comprehensive Guide to Coaching High School Cross Country, Running Fast, and Winning Championships

© 2022 Ken Sayles

Published in New York, New York, by Morgan James Publishing. Morgan James is a trademark of Morgan James, LLC. www.MorganJamesPublishing.com

Proudly distributed by Ingram Publisher Services.

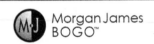

ISBN 9781631956133 paperback
ISBN 9781631956140 ebook
Library of Congress Control Number:
2021937298

Cover & Interior Design by:
Chris Treccani
www.3dogcreative.net

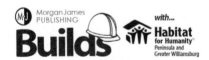

Morgan James is a proud partner of Habitat for Humanity Peninsula and Greater Williamsburg. Partners in building since 2006.

Get involved today! Visit MorganJamesPublishing.com/giving-back

This book honors my wonderful wife Melisa.

We met through running. We have run many miles together in some extraordinary places in the world. Her tireless and unselfish support of my coaching over almost thirty years is a constant source of inspiration to me. Being "Mrs. Coach" is not easy. The endless hours I spent buried in spreadsheets, and the time I spent on Saturdays at invitationals was time not spent with her. The amount of grace required for planning personal vacations and trips around my coaching schedule is a testament to how special a woman she is—a special wife. *Special*!

Thanks for always believing in me and supporting me.

TABLE OF CONTENTS

ACKNOWLEDGMENTS

I owe a great debt to many people for the time, wisdom, knowledge, and insight they have offered and the support they have shared and shown to me during my thirty-plus years as a cross country and track and field coach.

I thank my friend, the best man at my wedding, and a colleague and mentor, Tom White, for hiring me in 1987 at Capistrano Valley High in Mission Viejo, California, where I spent my coaching career.

Thanks to the many coaches that I shared with and learned from over all these years. I want to mention some special relationships I developed with my coaching colleagues:

To Randy Rossi, then of Irvine High, for those early years of conversations talking shop.

To Rich Medellin, of Esperanza High for thirty years of dialogue, comparing notes, and sharing joys and frustrations.

To Rex Hall, of Dana Hills High, for the shared love of the sport and his always generous sharing of workouts and wisdom.

To George Varvas, of Woodbridge High, for his inspiration and leadership over the years. His generous spirit and enthusiastic support when I finally got it right will always be appreciated.

Thanks to the many athletic directors and administrators who were so positive and supportive of our sport and my teams, especially Tom White, Tom Ressler, Christy Curtis, and Chad Addison.

To the extraordinary assistant coaches who did so much behind the scenes, as well as alongside me, to bring Capistrano Valley runners to the pinnacle of success.

Thanks to Shauna Herberg, Kristi Licata, and Patrick Corsinita for the wonderful pictures of the runners and teams in action.

To my wife, Melisa, for the hours spent editing this work.

To V. Tse-Horiuchi, for her help with formatting.

To coaching colleagues Dennis Kelly, Bob Price, and George Varvas, who took the time to read the manuscript and offer suggestions. To longtime friend and colleague Dr. Bill Hoffman who read thoroughly and edited wisely. To former runner and now young lawyer, Melissa Bell, who brought her usual attention to detail and lawyerly skills to a thorough edit.

To my agent Michael Ebeling. I could not have gotten this far without your wise counsel.

To David Hancock and Jim Howard at Morgan James Publishing—thanks for believing in me.

To the Author Support Team of Taylor Chaffer, Amber Parrott, Jessica Burton-Moran, and Heidi Nickerson, your assistance was remarkable. And to Emily Madison, my author relations manager, thank you for keeping everything organized and moving forward.

Thanks to my editor, Cortney Donelson, whose skill in copyediting and formatting was invaluable.

To the amazing parents who gave so selflessly and abundantly of their time, resources, and talents to help me develop, nurture, and care for their young athletes. There are too many to mention by name here, but "Thank You!"

Finally, to the athletes. I have had the wonderful experience of hearing from many of you over the years regarding your experience as a Capo Cougar. It is thrilling and humbling to realize the impact we coaches have on you, and I am so happy that it was a positive and joyous experience that we shared.

FOREWORD

This book contains one of the most complete and significant contributions to cross-country training methods for the high school program. Ken's long tenure and significant success in California high school cross country has been put to work to create a valuable aid to the cross-country coach and runner alike. This aid is a set of individualized season-long training plans, a week-by-week season calendar, and a comprehensive explanation of the role of each stake-holder involved in a high school program (coaches, athletes, and parents), which can be employed to set up custom-designed workouts for runners of all abilities.

A continuing problem for coaches is setting up training schedules that are neither too hard nor too easy for the runners. The information given in this book solves this problem by giving workout schedules designed for each individual runner's ability. Most of the established forms of distance training are explained and addressed within the workouts listed. This will give the coach and runner a wide choice of workouts for their training programs.

This book should be as valuable an aid to the coach as the stopwatch itself. It clearly explains the science involved in each training method utilized for the development of the distance athlete. It addresses the pre-season (summer preparation phase), the early, the competitive, and the championship phases; it covers and summarizes the governing regulations expected of the student-athletes in a high school cross-country program and thoroughly explains the financial challenges facing high school cross-country coaches as offering solutions to these challenges. The author accomplishes these goals in a simple, enthusiastic, and friendly manner. I recommend this book to the beginning and experienced coach.

George Varvas, race director, Woodbridge Cross Country Classic (world's largest high school meet), coach of two former national high school record holders, Christine Babcock at 1600 meters and Bethan Knights at 2 miles, and coach of multiple California Southern Section Team champions in cross country and track and field

PREFACE

When I began *Coach, Run, Win,* my original goal was to create a roadmap for coaches to navigate an entire high school cross-country season from start to finish. I believe this book does that in a comprehensive yet concise way. Yet the book has much more to offer than just a guide for coaches.

The first part of the book is focused on how to run fast. I provide details of training methods and workouts, which I used to help individuals and teams achieve nationwide success. These includes details on the workouts that one runner executed to become a California State champion. The information can be used by any runner, regardless of age, gender, or school affiliation. The advice about cross training, weightlifting, injury prevention, and the mental approaches to better racing are essential for success in running for everyone. I have provided several case studies outlining specific athletes to provide inspiration for all runners. These stories of athletes starting from non-running backgrounds, overcoming race-day anxiety, or facing the challenges of health conditions have universal appeal and application.

The second part of the book takes coaches through the details of the organization and implementation of a championship program for a school or organization. Subjects include: how to get potential runners to participate, how to organize parent and community support, and how to best work with school administrators. The challenges of establishing a summer program and executing an elite training camp are also addressed. The all-important end-of-season awards and banquets are deconstructed. Since most coaches—and many parents—have to be involved in designing and setting up race courses and managing races, I have a chapter on that too. I conclude with chapters on transitioning from cross country to track and field, as well as a chapter on virtual coaching. The chapter on virtual coaching has some helpful website resources listed.

Coach, Run, Win is about many things. It is certainly about how to coach runners. It is definitely about running and how to excel at it. The winning part is about helping coaches, teams, and individuals through developing positive attitudes and technical training data to accomplish their goals, whether they are winning state championships or improving from a walk to a shuffle to competing in a race for the first time.

ON YOUR MARKS, RUNNERS SET, GO!

CHAPTER 1:

INTRODUCTION

S o you just got hired to teach mathematics, but you had to agree to coach the cross-country team, and you have *no* idea where to start. This book is for you! That is not to say that veterans will not find something new or different here, as well—I know you can. This book is also for runners of all ages and experience levels, not just for the high school runner. Anyone can use the workouts detailed in these chapters to improve their own running. As the Preface explains, and as you can see from the Table of Contents, the early chapters focus on runners and how to coach them to run fast and win. The chapters on how to organize and administer a running program follow. They are organized and presented as a season of training and racing would unfold, so a coach can use these chapters as a step-by-step guide to coaching, running, and winning.

I love running! I began running as an adult and became addicted, running over 70,000 miles, much of it alongside the athletes I was lucky enough to coach for thirty-three years. I ran twenty-three marathons and qualified for Boston sixteen times. There is nothing quite like the feeling of accomplishment at the end of a hard workout or race. As a teacher who was also a runner, becoming a coach of runners was a natural thing to do. I am so glad I did, for the hours spent working with young people and helping them succeed at this great sport were some of the best hours of my life.

This book is not an overly technical book, especially in the sections on training. I will refer to other books and articles you may explore for a more scientific approach. This book comes from my trials, errors, and experiments over the years and settling on the ones that seemed to work best for my teams. I attended many seminars and read lots of books and articles. I spent hours each season talking with fellow coaches about what worked and what did not. This book grew from all those readings and conversations. Hopefully, I have saved you as a coach or runner from a lot of that work and experimentation as well as from some of the mistakes I made.

My hope is that *Coach, Run, Win* is like a conversation we are having about cross country. You bought me a coffee and asked if I would answer some questions about how I did things. Here are the answers! You can also contact me through my website at www. coachrunwin.com.

Though I have coached male distance runners (including a CIF champion at 3200 meters) and served as the overall track and field head coach for both boys and girls, my primary focus has always been as a *girls'* cross-country coach and *girls'* distance coach at track and field. Where relevant, I have reemphasized this point. I believe the overall approach detailed here is relevant to coaching both genders.

I suggest that **coaching boys and girls *is* different.** If you coach both boys and girls, you can certainly have them do similar workouts, drills, and warmups. Your mental and tactical approach can be similar. However, they are different. My experience is that girls are very social and need the chance to talk, share, and support each other. They respond poorly to "old-school," loud, and aggressive coaching. They are just as tough physically as boys and just as competitive on race day. The way they need to be rewarded along the way requires a conscious and positive attitude.

CHAPTER 2:

COACHING WINNING RUNNERS

How to Run Fast

hesitated to write the title to this section. I was not sure whether to include the word *winning* or not. Would that make what follows seem too elitist? Would you be discouraged from following the plans, assuming they were only for elite runners? In Chapter 5 and Chapter 8, you will find tools, techniques, and approaches to the mental side of racing. Everyone needs to have their own measure of what winning means for them. As you will see, this system that I refer to as the "Cougar Way" individualizes workouts, paces, and goals for every member of your team or every individual runner, regardless of their abilities.

Here is a reminder that my specific examples of times, distances, and paces will refer to the female athletes I coached. The key **Training Paces (Table 1 in the Appendix)** will be for both genders.

This section on training is *not* a complex, scientific, technical dissertation on training methods. If you want to know the chemistry, physiology, and biology of the workouts, you can find them in other books and online resources. I am sharing what worked for me and my athletes. These workouts produced a California State champion, a Nike Cross Nationals (NXN) All American, two Footlocker All Americans, multiple CIF Southern Section champions, and over fifty league champions. These workouts produced three sub-17:00, three-mile female runners and ten sub-17:20 female runners. It also brought many lower-level runners to major personal bests, creating the most successful non-varsity teams in our area. *These workouts worked!*

I coached for over thirty years and tried many different approaches. I went to many clinics in Southern California and heard numerous great coaches and experts discuss various training methods and approaches. I talked shop with wonderful colleagues on a weekly basis for years, trying to find the right mix. Each year, I read new articles and books, looking for the latest edge I could get.

However, I ran into a standard trap that I would urge you to be conscious of—too many cooks spoil the soup. In this context, I mean that you cannot mix and match several different systems and approaches. I did that for too long. I always had good teams and individuals, sometimes particularly good, but in hindsight, I may have held some of them back because I often had too many elements built into the system. I was trying to do too many different—and often conflicting—training concepts. The result was that athletes were sometimes over-trained, not peaking well. They were tired when championship time came because we had done too much of too many different things. Eventually, I came up with my system, the Cougar Way. As with many coaches, my winding journey eventually led to the great Dr. Jack Daniels and his book *Running Formula*. For a data nut like me, his VDOT chart was coaching nirvana (**See Table 1**).

Combined with my finally clear vision of what worked and what did not, I had the tools to provide success for my athletes.

I am hopeful that the trial and error that my athletes and I endured will help you be efficient, not wasting time or too many seasons trying to find the right formula for training success.

I will begin the discussion of the details of the workouts with a look at the types of workouts I used and their purposes. Then, I will discuss the basic phases of training and the emphasis of each. This will be followed by a discussion of how to plan a season from start to finish (actually from finish to start).

I explain how to use Jack Daniels's VDOT system to target individual training goals for each athlete. **Appendix 1** contains a two-page explanation of the system that a coach can send to athletes and parents or individual runners can use for guidance.

Types of Workouts

Long Run:

This run is typically done on Saturdays and constitutes the longest distance done by the athletes during a week. The distance itself varies depending on the experience, skill level, and week of the training cycle. For beginners, early in the summer, it could be three to five miles, and for veteran and elite runners, it may be six to seven miles. Build the distances go up a mile or two each week over the first half to two-thirds of the training cycle. The long run becomes deemphasized when peaking and tapering begin. My female athletes peaked between eleven and twelve miles for top experienced runners. Newer, or perhaps less talented runners, would get to eight or nine miles at peak.

The pace varies, of course, and details of how to calculate goals will be covered later. The simplest explanation of pace is that it should be conversational. An athlete should be able to carry on a conversation for the duration of the run and not lose their breath. If out of breath, especially early, they are going too fast. In this general discussion, top female runners ran 7:00–7:50 pace, middle athletes 8:15–9:00, and slower runners 9:30–11:00. These runs are at peak distance in the seventy-to-ninety-minute range. If you want to learn the science of pacing, check other sources, books or online. Heart-rate-based training would have the long run pace in the 60–75 percent of maximum heart rate. The maximum heart rate is generally calculated as 205–.5x age.

The purpose of the long run is twofold. Physically, it builds more mitochondria cells, which transport oxygen and blood to the muscles. More mitochondria mean more oxygen and more endurance. This physical build-up is a necessary steppingstone to other workouts and other phases. Mentally, it develops toughness and confidence in the athletes. The longer they go past the racing distance of three miles, or a 5k, the more confident runners can be in being able to complete that distance.

Medium Distance Run:

As the name suggests, this run is more in the four-to-seven-mile range with a time of thirty-five to fifty-five minutes. The pace is similar to the long run. It could be a bit faster as long as it remains conversational for the runner. The purpose is also similar to the long run, both mentally and physically. This run is often done midweek, especially early in the training cycle.

Recovery Run

This run is done in the minutes immediately after the completion of a hard effort, often a speed or tempo workout. The day after a long run can also be a recovery run. These runs can vary from two to four miles and are also at conversational pace. The reality is that right after a particularly hard effort, the ideal pace might be a challenge. I always felt that if athletes could stay within fifteen to thirty seconds of the ideal recovery pace, they were doing fine. The times here may range from fifteen to thirty-five minutes.

Tempo Run:

This was *the* run in my training cycle. I attribute much of our success to this one workout! Tempo Runs occurred weekly for eight to ten weeks, beginning around the third week of coach-led practices in the summer (sixth week of the cycle, overall). The last two times it is used in combination with some speed work as a transition to more race-specific workouts. I show this in detail later. You may see this workout done in a variety of ways: two-mile intervals, continuous twenty-to-thirty-minute runs, one-mile intervals, or 1200 meters. I prefer 1000 meters. It is a very manageable distance both physically and mentally. It can be done in a fairly confined area, so you as a coach, can monitor it carefully. My runners started out with three or four x 1000 with between 1:00- and 1:30-minute rests, depending on ability and background (more on calculating this later). Eventually, top girls would do eight x1000.

The pace is key, and this is where the science contained in my adaptation of the Daniels VDOT chart (**Table 1**) is crucial. I show you how to pick out the correct pace for each runner. The paces are twenty-four to thirty seconds a mile over three mile/5k race pace over 82–87 percent of max heart rate. The rest between each 1000-meter interval is short to prevent full recovery, which is the desired training effect. These workouts were usually done on Mondays. The purpose of the workout is to increase the anaerobic or lactate threshold of the runners. The non-scientific explanation is that this is the crucial barrier between when a runner goes from aerobic to anaerobic, literally beginning to lose her or his breath! Done at correct paces over two months, this workout allows runners to race faster and longer and do shorter speed workouts with less rest and more volume at higher paces.

A brief story: In 2011 and 2012, I had begun to realize that I had started traditional race-specific speed work (6x800 meters, 12x400 meters) too early in the training cycle and too often. The result was that athletes were tired when it came to championship time. In 2012, CVHS had an extremely talented young team with a chance to get to the coveted California State Meet for the first time. I decided early on to use these Tempo 1000s and forego the traditional speed work referred to above. I did add in some short speed development (as will be discussed next), mainly just for the mechanics of foot turnover and the feel of running fast. At the second meet of the season, the huge Woodbridge Invitational, on a very flat and fast course, I wondered if my runners would have the speed to compete well. They did! We set what was, at that time, a school record for team time (one to five runners) averaging 17:40 for three miles and finished second to nationally-ranked Saugus High School! This is what the Tempo 1000s can do for you and your team!

Speed Development

As referred to above in the Tempo section, I began using speed development runs generally on Tuesdays, following the tempos on Mondays. The workout consisted of a ladder down (declining amounts of work), totaling seven minutes of work: a three-minute hard effort (3200 pace) with 1:30 rest, a two-minute hard effort (between 1600 and 3200 pace) with one minute rest, a one-minute effort (800 pace) with thirty seconds rest, finishing with two thirty-second all-out efforts with a thirty-second rest in between. A twenty-five-to-thirty-five-minute recovery run completed the workout. The workout was done on a measured grass surface. The distance covered was recorded for comparison week to week. (See **Appendix 2** for a formula chart.) The paces overall ended up being close to an athlete's current mile race pace or a bit faster.

Hills

It is cross country after all! Here in California, we do not have as many authentic cross-country courses as in other areas of the country. Our most famous course, Mount San Antonio College (Mt. Sac), home of the Mt Sac Invitational, is very hilly. The State Meet course at Woodward Park in Fresno is moderately hilly. I have read that exercise physiologists suggest that hill work is equal to strength and speed work. I have also found that doing relatively short hill repeats is excellent for building good running form early in the season. It is physiologically hard to run uphill with bad form. Uphill training helps the body be more efficient. It is important to have runners focus on not leaning too far forward and to use a good, aggressive arm swing to lift the legs. There are a variety of different ways to do hill workouts, and I have used them all. I prefer short hill repeats of thirty to forty-five seconds, repeated six to eight times early in the training cycle. During the summer, my runners often did middle distance and recovery runs on moderately hilly terrain. As training and endurance advanced, I liked to do longer repeats, usually by timed effort. We had a practice site where we could do a ladder down on hills of five minutes, four minutes, three minutes, two minutes, and one minute, for example. Those would-be hard efforts uphill with easy shuffling downhill for recovery.

A word about words! High Intensity Interval Training (**HIIT**) is a term often used today. Many online and streaming running and biking programs are using the term to indicate a workout that uses alternating hard efforts of various lengths and intensities with rest periods.

The speed development described above and the following race pace workouts would fit the definition of HIIT workouts.

Traditional Race Pace Workouts

Here, I am referring to a variety of workouts characterized by working at, or under, three-mile/5k race pace. Examples include 6x800 and 12x400, with equal rests. As reported earlier, I did too much of this too soon for many years, so let that be a warning to you. These workouts are hard and a couple of days of rest/recovery are necessary afterward. I have come to believe from research and experience that these workouts are productive for five to seven weeks but probably not much more, especially if you race frequently. They become too tiring.

Race Simulation Workouts

This is a type of workout done sometimes early in the training cycle to see what athletes' fitness levels are. They can be used later in peaking and tapering time for a high quality, low quantity work effort. These workouts are usually done below race pace with exceptionally long rests. Examples for early in the training cycle would be 4-6x400 at 1600 goal pace with two-to-three-minute rests. Later in the cycle, it could be 2x600 at 1600 pace, with ten-minute rests, or 3x500 at 800 pace with eight-minute rests.

Tempo/Speed Mix Workouts

I used these as my runners transitioned away from tempo work into traditional speed work. This workout retains some of the strength and anaerobic threshold qualities while beginning to work on race-specific speed. An example is a 400-race pace start, short rest, then 3x1000 at tempo pace, with short rests (1:00–1:30), then an 800 with equal rest (rest equals the time run), a 400 with equal rest, and a 200 with equal rest. I used these two to three times in the transition from phase two into phase three (upcoming discussion) of the training cycle.

Phases of Training

I view a season in four phases: Base Phase, Strength/Stamina Phase, Speed Phase, and Peaking/Tapering Phase. Each phase has a general length and specific workouts associated with it that should be emphasized and then phased out as transition to the next phase begins.

Some coaches and authors describe the phases in terms of a pyramid. On the bottom is, of course, the Base Phase. It is the longest phase, and it's definitely necessary to support the other phases that build upon it. You cannot just skip to speed workouts.

A runner who does so will not be able to do as much speed, and if they try to, they are likely to become fatigued, injured, or both. Each of the other three phases are built on top of one another, forming the pyramid.

Base Phase

For my program, this phase lasted about eight weeks. It began with the captain-led practices at the start of summer and then continued into the first five weeks of coach-led official summer training. Certainly, with appropriate concern for mileage buildup, this can last as many as twelve weeks, as long as the types of workouts do not become too intense. This phase is all about miles and minutes. The key workout is the long run, and second in importance is the medium run. All paces are aerobic. There can be some hills incorporated in the runs and perhaps a short hill session as discussed earlier.

Strength/Stamina Phase

This phase lasts six to eight weeks. The key workout here is the tempo run. The long runs continue and even peak in mileage during this phase. Hill workouts are incorporated once a week, and the speed development workouts are used following the tempo workouts. For my program, this period overlapped with the start of racing, so the challenge was to find time in the schedule to get all the workouts in. Races are a form of speed work. Look at them that way in the midst of weekly or monthly planning. Your team's total mileage per week probably peaks during this phase.

Speed Phase

This phase lasts four to six weeks. The long run may be shortened or excluded all together. Tempo mix workouts replace the tempo run. This is when traditional race pace workouts are done. The mileage per week should be declining as you are likely into racing mode. Begin some race simulation workouts here, as well.

Peaking/Tapering Phase

I have talked with many coaches over the years, and we all agree: this phase can be a mystery. There are many theories and much research done about what your team should and should not be doing to taper. I will share my approach with you and why I chose to do it this way. I took about three weeks to taper. Mileage came down perhaps 30–40 percent from peak. There were no long runs and no tempo runs. The speed work had to be high quality and low quantity with longer rests. Some authors and researchers suggest a radical reduction in mileage; others support a very minimal change in mileage. My approach struck a middle ground. The key is to maintain the intensity of workouts and watch rest and recovery so that the runners do not become stale. Distance runners like to run! Whether it is physiological or psychological, I found that too much tapering was not good for my runners.

Planning Your Season

First, you need to clearly establish the length of your season by deciding how far your team is going to go in terms of your particular championship scenarios. For an individual runner, you need to determine when your goal race will occur. As discussed, set your goals high, but be realistic. **You need to plan the start of your season and training by counting backward from the projected end of your season or goal race!** For my team, the State Meet was Thanksgiving weekend. So, we began tapering and peaking three weeks before the State Meet. This included our League Finals race and our two levels of regional qualifying (CIF Prelims and Finals) race. For four to six weeks prior to the tapering phase is the Speed Phase; for my team, that meant much of October. Then count back for the six to eight weeks of the Strength/Stamina Phase, which goes backward through September into early August. The Base Phase then, depending on your area's rules about contact and your own choices for the summer, will begin somewhere in June.

A word about the mix of workouts. Much has also been studied and written about the right mix of types of workouts. That is, what percentage or how much mileage should be devoted to each of the types of workouts in each phase. In the Base Phase, almost one hundred percent of the running is aerobic. In the Strength/Stamina Phase, about 80–85 percent is aerobic, and 8–10 percent is tempo, with 2–3 percent speed development. In the Speed Phase, 70–75 percent is still aerobic, but 10–15 percent is speed, and 2–3 percent is speed development and tempo. Finally, in the Peaking/Tapering Phase 60–70 percent is aerobic, 15–25 percent is speed, and 4–6 percent is speed development.

This calculation should be based on your own view of how much mileage you are comfortable having your athletes run at any one time. For example, in the Strength/ Stamina Phase, as a mid-mileage coach, I may have had my athletes running forty to sixty miles per week (with top female athletes in the fifty-five to sixty range). So roughly forty to forty-five miles were aerobic (that includes warmup and warm down) and about four to five miles were tempo workouts. I spent a lot of time calculating this and worrying about it for years. Races complicate the situation. How do you calculate and classify races? Next, I will show you the specific workout week examples that are the result of experiments, as well as my own experience in answering that question.

Designing Individual Workout Goals for Each Member of Your Team

What I am about to describe can be very labor intensive. However, it is absolutely necessary to make this system work for each athlete from fastest to slowest. Use assistant coaches, injured athletes, team managers, aides, and helpful parents as data gatherers and number crunchers. It can be done. I began this protocol and maintained it year-round for track and field, as well, while teaching Advanced Placement (AP) Government and IB History of the Americas full-time. The success your athletes and teams will achieve makes the effort more than worthwhile.

Beginning in the summer with the earliest workouts, record distances, times, and paces for each athlete. Once you have two weeks of workouts recorded, begin to individualize the workouts. I adapted Jack Daniels's Table, "Training Intensities Associated with Current VDOT," to one page (See **Table 1**) for easy use with the distances my team would likely train at and the VDOTs they would likely be assigned.

Jack Daniels wrote *Daniels Running Formula,* in which he presents his VDOT system. Dr. Daniels has a Doctoral Degree in Exercise Physiology. He measured, tested, and studied thousands of runners over many years. His research combines heart rate, VO2 max, and other measurements of fitness to arrive at his VDOT system. His complex, technical, scientific studies were simplified in **Table 1** to provide an accurate way of telling athletes how fast to run in any given workout to maximize their individual development. Daniels has taken the guesswork out of determining at what paces athletes should run. Instead of saying, "run at 80 percent," or "run hard," it is possible to give each runner a specific pace that matches their current abilities and level of fitness. I have summarized this on one page for easy reference (**Table 1**).

After you have gathered the initial data about distance, time, and pace, find the average pace of those runs in the E pace column on my "Training Paces" (**Table 1**).

Then look to the far left and find the VDOT associated with that pace. This is the initial VDOT for the athlete. Do this for each one of your athletes. Continue to record the data (distance, time, pace) for all subsequent workouts, and then adjust VDOTs as workouts and training progress. For cross country, the most frequently used categories are the E pace for long, medium, and recovery runs. I paces are basically race-pace speed workouts, and T is for tempo. R paces are near 1600 pace, so use them for under cross-country pace-speed work. F paces are intended for track and field.

For any given workout, from the long run to the recovery run and on into tempo workouts and various speed work, simply find the pace indicated for a given workout distance and type what corresponds to an athlete's individual VDOT. For example, for an athlete with a VDOT of 50, preparing for a Tempo 1000 workout, look at T paces 1000. Then see the paces associated for this athlete are 4:14. I would prepare a goal sheet (See **Resources** for a sample) for the workout with each athlete listed, their goal, and provide empty spaces to record each interval completed. An injured athlete or assistant coach can help gather this data.

I regularly emailed the results of the workouts to athletes and parents. Athletes are held accountable and responsible by seeing documentation of how they are doing. Hopefully, it inspires them to do their best. Parents also receive this information, which has several benefits: It helps them to see, believe in, and support the technical sophistication of the training system, and they support and motivate their athletes in positive ways by seeing the results.

CHAPTER 3:

A CHAMPIONSHIP SEASON

One Workout at a Time

From 2012 to 2018, I decided that our team goal was to make it into the California State Championship Race held Thanksgiving weekend. I counted backward twenty-three weeks from State Meet race day to establish the beginning of athlete-led practices. The beginning of official coach-led summer practice began in mid-July. The Base Phase, emphasizing long runs, started with captain/athlete-led practices and lasted eight to nine weeks. The Strength/Stamina Phase, emphasizing the tempo runs and hill work, lasted about seven to eight weeks. The Speed Phase, emphasizing race-specific speed work lasted four to five weeks, and the Peaking/Tapering Phase had a duration of three weeks.

Slow but steady buildup of miles was imperative as I previously emphasized. Captain-led practices were held three to four times a week with mileage accumulating from a starting point of fifteen to twenty-five miles, which included the warmup at each practice. The goal was for runners to get to approximately twenty-five to thirty-five miles by the time coach-led practices began in mid-July. The assumption was that runners had, in fact, done the prescribed work and therefore could start as indicated in the detailed section that follows. Please remember that the miles totals are reflective of **female runners**. Each workout should begin with a dynamic warmup, which consisted of ten to twenty minutes of running (my preference was twelve minutes) followed by active drills and exercises to specifically prepare for the workout. A stretch down should follow the run. (See **Resources** for a Warmup and Warm-down.) I have also included a wonderful Practice Etiquette handout created by Capistrano Valley Boys' Coach Matt Soto (**Appendix 3**). A Pace, Distance, and Miles Chart is referenced in the **Resources** and can be found on my website.

Phase 1: Base Phase

Runners had spent three weeks building base through captain-led weeks.

Week Four Overall (Week One of Coach-Led)

Remember to record as much data as possible to help determine paces using **Table 1** (explained earlier).

Monday:
- 40–45-minute medium distance run.

Tuesday:
- Discuss form, rhythmic breathing, stride frequency, and shoe-tying (see Chapter 7: Tricks of the Trade).
- Speed Development—Flying 40s 4x (20-meter build-up, 40-meter all-out, 20-meter slow-down) and 30-minute recovery run.

Wednesday:
- 40–45-minute medium distance run.

Thursday:

- Hill Workout—teach hill technique (see Chapter 7: Tricks of the Trade), continuous hill run for veterans and short hill repeats for newcomers.

Friday:

- Workout on own without team—cross train, rest, or pool work.

Saturday:

- 50–55-minute long run.

Sunday:

- Rest or cross train for no more than 30 minutes.

Total miles for week with 1–1.5-mile warmups included: 27–38 miles.

Week Five Overall (Week Two of Coach-Led)

Remember to record data.

Monday:

- 40–45-minute medium distance run.

Tuesday:

- Discuss form, rhythmic breathing, stride frequency, and shoe-tying
  Speed Development-Flying 40s 6x (20-meter build-up, 40-meter all-out, 20-meter slow-down) and 30-minute recovery run.

Wednesday:

- 45–50-minute Medium Distance Run.

Thursday:

- Hill repeat loops of two to three minutes, 20-minute recovery run, review technique.

Friday:

- Water/Pool running, if available.

Saturday:

- Long run for 55–60 minutes.

Sunday:

- Rest or cross train for no more than 30 minutes.

Total miles for week with 1–1.5-mile warmups included: 27–38 miles.

Week Six Overall (Week Three of Coach-Led)

Monday:

- Tempo 1000s—use data collected to establish goal times as discussed previously; depending on size of team, suggest three groups doing 4, 5, or 6 x1000 at T pace with 1:15, 1:30, and 1:45 rests for the three groups, 15–20-minute cool-down.

Tuesday:

- Speed Development—review form, stride frequency, breathing, 7-min speed ladder, and 25-minute recovery.

Wednesday:

- 50–55-minute medium distance run.

Thursday:

- Hill Run 45–55 minutes on continuous hilly surface, review hill technique.

Friday:

- Pool work, if able or cross train or short recovery run for 25–30 minutes.

Saturday:

- Long run for 55–60 minutes with effort to be faster than previous Saturday.

Sunday: Rest.

Total miles for week at practice with the 1–1.5 warm up included: 33–45 miles.

Two-A-Days

At this point in the summer, I encouraged but did not require a second practice once or twice a week in the early evening. This was designed to add miles and minutes to the totals and stimulate the body to rebuild muscle. Doing two-a-days is a common practice for many programs in the summertime when school is not in session. Some coaches do two-a-days just one day a week; some do more. Certainly, there can be a point at which you are adding too much work and not leaving enough time to promote recovery and rest. Where that point is may be a function of your overall workload and your philosophy of mileage.

Mileages I show from here on out, *do* include one extra workout. Mileages would be up about 4-6 miles a week with just one day of the extra workouts.

Week Seven Overall (Week Four of Coach-Led)
Monday:
- Tempo 1000s 5, 6, or 7 with 1:10, 1:25, and 1:40 rests by group with 20–25-minute recovery.

Tuesday:
- Review teaching items from previous Tuesdays—6xFlying 40s, 30-minute recovery.

Wednesday:
- 50–55-minute medium distance run.

Thursday:

- Hill work—pyramid by time. For example, 30 seconds, 45 seconds, 1 minute, 1:30, 1 minute, 45 seconds, 30 seconds, with 20–25-minute recovery.

Friday:

- Pool work or 30–35-minute recovery run.

Saturday:

- Long run for 60–65 minutes.

Sunday:

- Rest or cross train, no more than 30 minutes.

Total miles for week at practice with 1–1.5-mile warmup with a two-a-day: 37–53 miles.

Week Eight Overall (Week Five of Coach-Led)

Monday:

- Tempo 1000s 5, 6, or 7 with 1:00, 1:15, and 1:30 rests by group with 15–20-min recovery.

Tuesday:

- Speed ladder, 7 min and 30-minute recovery.

Wednesday:

- 50–55 medium distance run.

Thursday:

- Continuous hill run for 40–50 minutes.

Friday:

- Water running, rest, or core work.

Saturday:

- Long run for 65–70 minutes.

Sunday:

- Rest or cross train, no more than 35 minutes.

Total miles at practice with 1–1.5-mile warmup included and a two-a-day: 37–51 miles.

This is the time period where the invite-only Mammoth Lakes camp would occur. Those invited athletes would be doing two-a-days for several days and adding fifteen to twenty miles to weekly totals (for fifty to sixty miles a week) over a number of weeks.

Phase Two: Strength/Stamina Phase

Week Nine Overall (Week Six of Coach-Led)
Monday:
- Tempo 1000s 5–7 with 1:00, 1:10, 1:20 rests by group with 20–25-minute recovery.

Tuesday:
- Downhill technique practice (5–7 x60–100-meter downhills on grass or dirt) 6 flying 40s, and 25–30-minute recovery.

Wednesday:
- 45–50-minute recovery run.

Thursday:
- Hill repeats 8–10 35–45-second uphill with downhill shuffle, 25–30-minute recovery.

Friday:
- 45–50-minute recovery run.

Saturday:
- Long run for 65–75 minutes.

Sunday:
- Rest or cross train, no more than 35 minutes.

Total miles with warmup included and one two-a-day: 39–54.

Week Ten Overall (Week Seven of Coach-Led)
Monday:
- Tempo 1000s 5–7 with 1, 1:10, 1:20 rests by group 20–25-min-ute recovery.

Tuesday:

- Speed development, downhills as in week nine, 7-minute speed ladder.

Wednesday:

- 50–60-minute-long recovery run.

Thursday:

- Hill loops, longer 4–6 x 2–4-minute repeats on hilly terrain and 20–25-minute recovery.

Friday:

- Pool work or 30–35-minute recovery run.

Saturday:

- Long run for 70–80 minutes.

Sunday:

- Rest or cross train.

Total miles with warmup and one two-a-day: 40–57 miles.

Week Eleven Overall (Week Eight of Coach-Led)

Monday:

- Tempo 1000s 6–8 with 1:10, 1:20, 1:30 rests and 20–25-minute recovery.

Tuesday:

- Speed development, downhills, 8 Flying 40s, and 30-minute recovery.

Wednesday:

- 50–60-minute-long recovery run.

Thursday:

- Short hill repeats and 25–30-minute recovery.

Friday:

- 30–35-minute recovery run.

Saturday:

- Long run for 70–80 minutes. This would be our beach run and team meeting with parents described in a Chapter 13, the week before our first meet.

Sunday: Rest.

Total miles with warmup and one two-a-day: 40–57 miles.

Week 12 begins the first of our Saturday Invitational Meets—I am going to show this part of the training as if that were your case as well. My program did not continue with two-a-days.

Week Twelve Overall (Week Nine of Coach-Led)
Monday:

- Tempo 1000s 6–8 with 1:10, 1:20, 1:30 rests, 20–25-minute recovery.

Tuesday:

- Speed development, short downhill practice, 7-minute ladder, 30-minute recovery.

Wednesday:

- 50–60-minute-long recovery.

Thursday:

- Short hill repeats with 25–30-minute recovery.

Friday:

- PRE-MEET—see section to follow regarding pre-meet workouts, meeting, and goal setting.

Saturday:

- Invitational Race—usual warmup routine, 25–30-minute cool-down after race.

Sunday:

- 20–30-minute recovery run.

Total miles for week: 38–53 with warmups.

Week Thirteen Overall (Week Ten of Coach-Led)

The order shifts due to the race the previous Saturday.

Monday:

- Speed development, 7-minute pyramid (30 seconds, 1 minute, 2 minutes, 2 minutes, 1 minute, 30 seconds with 30, 30 1, 1, 30 rests, short downhill practice, 30-minute run.

Tuesday:

- Long run for 55–65 minutes.

Wednesday:

- Tempo 1000s 6–8x1000 with 1:00, 1:10, 1:20 rests and 20–25-minute recovery.

Thursday:

- 45-minute recovery run.

Friday: Pre-meet.

Saturday: Invitational Race.

Sunday:

- Cross train or 20–25-minute recovery run.

Total miles for week: 38–53 with warmups.

Week Fourteen Overall (Week Eleven of Coach-Led)

(Extra work because no meet this week.)

Monday:

- Long run for 65–70 minutes.

Tuesday:

- Tempo 1000s 6–8 same rests as Week Thirteen.

Wednesday:

- Medium recovery run for 45 minutes.

Thursday:

- Long hill repeats, ladder down 4 minutes, 3 minutes, 2 minutes, 1 minute with shuffle. Recovery with shuffle downhill, recovery between each interval.

Friday: Pre-meet.

Saturday: Invitational Race.

Sunday:

- Cross train, rest, or 25-minute recovery run.

Total miles for week: 40–52 miles with warmups.

Week Fifteen Overall (Week Twelve of Coach-Led)

(Begins transition to Phase Three)

Monday:

- Long run for 65–70 minutes (longest remaining long run).

Tuesday:

- Tempo and speed mix 400 race start, 1:30 rest, 4 or 5x Tempo 1000 with 1:10 rests 800 at race pace with 2:30 rest, 400 race finish and 20-minute recovery.

Wednesday:

- Medium recovery run for 45 minutes.

Thursday:

- Short hill repeats 8–10x, 40 seconds and 25–30-minute recovery.

Friday:

- Speed development, downhill practice, 6x flying 40s, 30-minute recovery.

Saturday:

- Long run for 60–70 minutes.

Sunday: Rest.

Total miles for week: 38–52 with warmups.

Phase Three: Speed

Week Sixteen Overall (Week Thirteen of Coach-Led)
A unique week for my teams due to League meet on Tuesday and travel invitational for Top 12 on Saturday.

Monday: Pre-meet.

Tuesday: League races.

Wednesday:

- 40–45-minute recovery.

Thursday:

- Long hill ladder (4, 3, 2, 1 minutes) with 20–25-minute recovery.

Friday:

- Pre-meet for Top 12, long run for rest of team.

Saturday:

- Invitational for Top 12, rest, or cross train day for rest of the team.

Sunday:

- Rest for majority of team, cross train, or 25-minute recovery run for those at Invitational.

Total miles for week: 25–33 for non-Saturday racers, 35–40 miles for Saturday racers.

Week Seventeen Overall (Week Fourteen of Coach-Led)
Saturday was the big regional Orange County Championship Race. I begin to split the group for many of the workouts into those likely to be ending their seasons at League Finals in three weeks to a month and those likely to be a part of the post-season team going on, hopefully another six weeks, which was about ten to twelve runners.

Group 1 going six weeks, the CIF/Championship team

Group 2 finishing the season in three to four weeks

Monday:

- Group 1—Long run for 60–65 minutes.
- Group 2—Speed work, tempo 1000 with 1:30 rest, 4x800 at race pace with two-minute rest, 2x400 at sub-race pace (R in Training Pace chart) with 1:30 rests, 15–20-minute recovery run.

Tuesday:

- Group 1—Speed tempo mix 400 race; start with 1:30 rest, 2xTempo 1000 w/ one-minute rest, 800 at race pace with 2:30 rest, 2xTempo 1000 with one-minute rest, 300, 200 fast pace, with 20-minute recovery run.
- Group 2—Speed development day, downhills, 6x60, and 30-minute recovery run.

Wednesday:

- Group 1—Medium distance recovery for 45 minutes.
- Group 2—Speed work, three sets of 400 sub-race pace with two minutes rest, 800 at race pace with three-minute rest, 400 all out to finish, 20-minute recovery.

Thursday:

- Group 1—Speed ladder, 7-minute version, and 30-minute recovery run
- Group 2—40-minute recovery run.

Friday: Pre-meet.

- Saturday: Orange County Championships Invitational Race.
- Sunday: Rest, cross train, or 20-minute recovery options.

Total miles for the week for Group 1: 40–46 and Group 2: 30–36.

Week Eighteen Overall (Week Fifteen of Coach-Led)

Mt. Sac Invitational Week

Monday:

- Group 1—Long recovery run for 55–60 minutes.
- Group 2—Medium recovery run for 40–45 minutes.

Tuesday:

- Speed/hill combination (held base of a hill) so flat speed before an uphill section, simulate Mt. Sac course 800, 600, 400 with 2:30 shuffles and 25-minute recovery run.

Wednesday:

- Group 1—Medium distance recovery run for 45 minutes
- Group 2— Medium distance recovery run for 35 minutes

Thursday:

- All Speed Development, downhills, 7-minute speed ladder, and 20–25-minute recovery run.

Friday: Pre-meet.

Saturday:

- Invitational Race (Mt. Sac Invitational)

Sunday:

- Rest for Group 2, if healthy 20-minute recovery run for Group 1.

Total miles for the week for Group 1: 40–45 miles and Group 2: 30–35 miles.

Week Nineteen Overall (Week Sixteen of Coach-Led)

Monday: Recovery run

- Group 1—45–55 minutes
- Group 2—40–45 minutes with 2x300 finishes.

Tuesday: Speed work

- Group 1—400 start, 1:30 rest, 3xTempo 1000 with one-minute rest, 800 at race pace with 2:30 rest, 400 at race pace or under with 1:30 rest 400 fast, and 20-minute recovery run.
- Group 2—Pyramid all at sub race pace (R on Training Pace chart **Table 1**), 300, 1-minute rest, 400, 2-minute rest, 600, 3-minute rest, 800, 3-minute rest 600, 3-minute rest, 400, 2-minute rest, 300 all out, and 15–20-minute recovery.

Wednesday:

- 40–45-minute recovery run with 300, 200 fast finish simulations.

Thursday: Speed work.

- Group 1—Speed/hill combo, an uphill section, (Mt. Sac course) 800, 600, 400 with 2:30 shuffles in between, 25-minute recovery run.
- Group 2—8x400 at sub-race pace (R on chart) with 2-minute rests and 15–20-minute recovery run.

Friday:

- 30–35-minute recovery run.

Saturday:

- Long run with focus on pace at fastest edge of appropriate pace or negative split
- Group 1—50–55 minutes
- Group 2—40–45 minutes.

Sunday: Rest.

Total miles for week Group 1: 43-50 miles, group 2 :30-37 miles

Week Twenty Overall (Week Seventeen of Coach-Led)

Monday:

- Speed work both groups 6x400 at sub race pace with 2:30–3-minute rests, 20–25-minute recovery run.

Tuesday: Pre-meet.

Wednesday: League Finals races.

Thursday:

- 40–45-minute recovery run.

Friday:

- Post-season team only from now on, speed work 7-minute ladder with 25-minute recovery.

Saturday:

- Long run for 60–65 minutes.

Sunday: Rest.

Total miles for week: 31–41 miles.

Phase Four: Peaking and Tapering Phase

Week Twenty-One Overall (Eighteen of Coach-Led)

Just CIF/Championship team

Monday:

- 40–45-minute hill run with 2x200 practice, all-out finishes.

Tuesday:

- Speed work, 400 race start, 3xTempo 1000 with 1-minute rests, 800 at race pace with 2:30 rest, 400 at race pace, 2-minute rest, 200 all-out and 25-minute recovery.

Wednesday:

- 40–45-minute recovery run.

Thursday:

- Speedwork pyramid 300, 400, 600, 600, 400, 300 all sub-race pace with rests of 1, 1:30, 2, 2, 1:30 minutes each with 20-minute recovery run.

Friday: Pre-meet.

Saturday:

- CIF Prelims (first round of playoffs in Southern Section of CIF in California).

Sunday:

- Optional 30-minute recovery run.

Total miles for week: 37–40 miles with the race.

Week Twenty-Two Overall (Week Nineteen of Coach-Led)

Monday:

- Speed work 6x400 at R or sub-race pace with 3-minute rests, 25-minute recovery run

Tuesday:

- 35–40-minute recovery run with flying 40s (4–6).

Wednesday:

- Speed work, 7-minute ladder.

Thursday:

- 30–35-minute recovery run.

Friday: Pre-meet.

Saturday:

- CIF Finals for Southern Section qualifying to go to State Meet.

Sunday: rest.

Total miles for week: 28–35 with race.

Week Twenty-Three Overall (Week Twenty of Coach-Led)

STATE CHAMPIONSHIP WEEK in California

Monday:

- 35–40-minute recovery run.

Tuesday:

- Speed work, 400 race start, 2-minute rest, tempo 1000 1-minute rest, 800 at race pace, 3-minute rest, 400, 300, 200 with 2:00, 1:30 and 1:00-minute rests, 20-minute recovery run.

Wednesday:

- 30-minute recovery run.

Thursday:

- 25-minute recovery run and 2x200 finishes.

Friday:

- Travel and pre-meet at State Meet site—Woodward Park, Fresno, California.

Saturday: California State Championships.

Sunday: Rest.

Total miles for week: 24–30 with race.

CASE STUDY: HALEY HERBERG
The Making of a State Champion

Haley began her storied career at Capistrano Valley High School in the summer of 2014.

She had been around the program for several years since her older sister Natalie (see her own case study) had just graduated. Haley had recently won the 1500 meters at the USTAF national championships, so expectations were high for her impact on our program. She joined a team that had already made the State Championships two years in a row, and Haley helped them to a 2nd place finish at State and a number eight national ranking.

As a freshman, Haley ran a season best of 17:47. During her sophomore year, she lowered that time to 17:12 while helping to lead the team to another State Championship finals race. During her junior year, she clearly established herself as one of California's—and the nation's—best runners. She lowered her best time to 16:46 while leading the Cougars to another State Final. She won the first of two South Coast League and two Orange County individual titles.

Haley's best was yet to come when her senior year produced a personal best of 16:01. She set several course and meet records on the way to compiling a career record of five races under 16:45, ten races under 17:06, and twenty-seven races under eighteen minutes. She finished her remarkable career with a dominating performance in the post season, winning CIFSS and State titles by wide margins—the latter in a historic 17:00 minutes for 5k on the storied Woodward Park, Fresno, California course. This earned her an invite as an individual to NXN where she achieved All-American status.

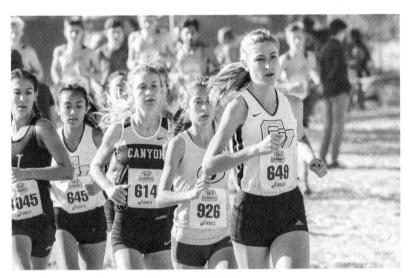

Haley leading at Finals

She would begin her college career at the University of Oklahoma before transferring to the University of Washington where she is helping the Huskies to elite team status. In March 2021, she won the COVID-delayed 2020 Pac-12 Cross Country Championship!

Before detailing how she did this, a word about her track and field accomplishments is in order. If you would like to see details of her track and field workout in 2017, see my website at www.coachrunwin.com. Haley would compile personal bests of 4:47.55 for 1600, 10:09.54 for 3200, and three California State Meet finals in track and field and CIFSS individual championship at 1600 meters.

Haley brought remarkable physical attributes to her distance-running career. She was tall and strong with long strides that ate up the ground before her. She was relatively injury free, a result of her attention to caring for her body and the good fortune of a strong genetic makeup. (Her parents were both college runners). She was exceptionally good about communicating with me when she needed some rest.

Mentally, Haley was very disciplined and extremely focused. She loved to compete but was not overly stressed by it. She brought a phenomenal dedication to her workouts, and it showed in the consistency of her race performances. Haley loved race planning with me and coming to an agreement on her goals and tactics for each race. She was extremely coachable, which made our relationship even more enjoyable.

Here is a brief overview of sample weeks from her 2017 State Championship season:

- **Mid-August**
  Monday: 7x1000 at tempo pace (3:33) with 1:10 rests
  Tuesday: a 7-minute speed ladder of 3 minutes, 2 minutes, 1 minute, and 2 30-second intervals, which covered 1.35 miles in her case or roughly 5:20 pace
  Wednesday: 60-minute recovery run of about 8 miles
  Thursday: Long hill repeats of 4 minutes, 3 minutes, 2 minutes, 1 minute
  Friday: 40-minute recovery run or around 5.5 miles
  Saturday: Long run of 11 miles at 7:10 pace
- **Mid-September (following a Saturday Invitational race)**
  Monday: 45-minute recovery run of 6 miles
  Tuesday: Long run of 9.5 miles at 7:10 pace
  Wednesday: 8x1000 at tempo pace (3:30) with 1:10 rests
  Thursday: 7-minute speed ladder (see Tuesday above)
  Friday: Pre-meet
  Saturday: Invitational race with 25–30-minute cool-down
  Sunday: 25–30-minute recovery run on her own
- **Mid-October (two key invitationals, Orange County and Mt. Sac)**
  Monday: Long run of 65 minutes, around 9 miles at 7:10 pace
  Tuesday: 400 race start, 7x1000 tempo pace (under 3:30) and 400 race finish
  Wednesday: 45-minute recovery run, around 6.5 miles
  Thursday: Speed ladder as above
  Friday: Pre-meet

Saturday: Orange County Champs (a second win), Mt. Sac (3rd in 17:05)

Sunday: 25–30-minute recovery run on own

- **Early November (League Finals and CIFSS prelims)**

    Monday: 8x400 at 1:15 or 400 start, 7x1000 tempo at 3:28, 400 finish at 1:13

    Tuesday: 40–45-minute recovery 5.5–6 miles

    Wednesday: Pre-meet or speed pyramid 300 at :53, 400 at 1:14, 600 at 1:56, 800 at 2:35, 600 at 1:57, 400 at 1:13, 300 at :53

    Thursday: League finals or 40-minute recovery

    Friday: 40-minute recovery or pre-meet

    Saturday: Long run of 60 minutes at 7:05 pace or CIF Prelims (won heat, 17:24 casual, not all-out effort)

    Sunday: 20-minute recovery run

- **CIFSS Finals week**

    Monday: 45 minutes at 7:10 pace

    Tuesday: 400 at 1:15, 3x1000 tempo at 3:28 pace, 600 at 1:58, 400 at 1:14, 200 at :34

    Wednesday: 35-minute recovery at 7:20 pace

    Thursday: 40 minutes at 7:20 pace

    Friday: pre-meet

    Saturday: *CIFSS Finals won in meet and course record of 16:24*

- **California State Championships week**

    Monday: 45-minute recovery run 6 miles

    Tuesday: 400 at 1:14, 3x1000 tempo at 3:28 pace, 600 at 1:57, 400 at 1:14, 200 at :33

    Wednesday: Speed ladder (see above)

    Thursday: 35-minute recovery run for 4.5 miles

    Friday: Pre-meet

    Saturday: California State Champion, Division 2 *in 17:00 for hilly 5k, Top 10 time, all time*

CHAPTER 4:

RACING

How to Win with Techniques, Strategies, and Tactics

The training and preparation are ongoing. Now it is time to put it all on the line. It is Race Day! I will cover a number of topics: scoring, racing techniques, goal setting, the practicalities of race day warmup, and more. The mental approach to racing successfully will be covered in the next

chapter.

Scoring

Cross-country races are scored by adding up the finishing places of the top five runners on the team. The lowest score wins. In the event of a tie, the team with the fastest sixth person wins. This is something to stress to all members of a team. Every runner may count. Another thing to emphasize, which will keep more than just the top five or six runners motivated and alert to their positions, is displacement. Displacement happens when a team's non-scoring runners finish ahead of another team's scoring runners. This is where depth on a team can really make a difference.

Racing Tactics and Strategies

There are several tactics that can be executed over the course of a cross-country race to help improve the team score.

Packing

Packing is when several team members are close enough together during a race to prevent members of other teams from getting between them. When packing occurs, it can raise the score of the opposition teams. For example, when Team A finishes one, four, five, six, and seven, and Team B finishes two, three, eight, nine, and ten, then A's pack of four, five, six, and seven, blocks out B's scorers. Each time a runner passes a scorer from another team, it causes a two-point swing—so one point less for Team A and one more point for team B. This effect is multiplied by packing.

Can packing be practiced? I once asked a friend and colleague, George Varvas, how he got one of his many excellent teams to pack so well on race day. He laughed heartily and said it only happened on race day. No matter what he tried to do at practice, the runners spread out too much.

I suspect George was being a bit modest here, but in reality, it is hard to get runners with different work ethics and abilities to run close together during practice. However, I found that using groupings based on the VDOT system helps with packing since runners with similar abilities are grouped together.

Surging

A standard in-race tactic is to speed up, or surge, for a brief time (five to thirty seconds). The surge accomplishes two things. First, it tests the competitive resolve of the nearest competitors. Secondly, if done mid-race, surging helps to keep the runners' pace from slowing down, which inevitably occurs from fatigue and lack of mental focus.

Surging can be practiced in several ways during different practice runs. On a distance run, runners can be directed to surge at random, at specified intervals, and for various lengths of time. I have also used a game/gimmick called "blind surges." Runners draw slips of paper with a specified surge time and order of placement. Each runner keeps her/his information secret. Several minutes into the run, whoever drew surge *number one* executes the surge assigned to them for the time designated on the paper. *Number two* waits for a few minutes (however long you designate) and decides to execute her/his surge. This surge practice forces runners to be aware of others and respond to competitors' actions.

Speed workouts can also be used for surge practice. Use a whistle, horn, or voice commands to direct surges for various lengths of time. A specific interval can also be designated as a surge interval, where runners go faster than they normally would for that distance or specific length of time.

Course Management

When possible, practicing on the actual race courses is especially important. It provides essential knowledge of how to physically run a particular race. Where are the hills? Where are the blind corners for a surprise surge? Where is the mile mark? That knowledge of the physical layout and understanding of how to manage it, provide important mental preparedness and confidence. Try to hold several summer practices at the site of the first meet. Do drills, cool-downs, and stretch down in the actual places where the race will take place. The familiarity is immensely powerful. It helps calm nerves, especially for first timers. Provide all runners with a physical map of the course so they can trace through it and visualize the race. Provide photos of the course if you can. These should include the start and finish areas, key turns, and the mile markers.

Pre-Race or Pre-Meet Workout

There are many ways to design the last workout prior to a race. Some coaches have their runners do a large amount of work, especially early in the season. They argue that it helps build strength and stamina for the championship season to come. Other coaches emphasize the mental side of helping the runners mini-peak and feel fresh for the race the next day. An appropriate middle ground in terms of balancing the mental demands with the physical is my preference.

We would start with our normal warmup routine. Then we would practice some starts of 200–300 meters. I instructed runners how to line up at the start line in a tight group to maximize the opportunity of them getting out ahead of slower starters. It is important to teach and practice the start exactly as it will happen in the upcoming race. If the race implements a single-file start, practice that. If the start allows two or three across, practice that. The runners will be less nervous and more confident once they have experienced the simulated race start.

Next, we did a twenty-to-twenty-five-minute cool-down run before the usual stretch down. Finally, the team meeting took place if we had not done it before practice. Late in the season and at championship time, the cool-down was shortened to fifteen to twenty minutes.

Pre-Meet Dinner

This is a fun team-building activity that can be done in a number of ways.

The Booster parents worked awfully hard to provide a pasta party for one hour the night before most of the races. A simple meal of pasta, various sauces, salad, bread, and fluids was provided. Our dinners combined the boys' and girls' teams. Note: Research shows that carb-loading really does not help much for distances below the half marathon distance (13.1 miles) so this is simply a ritual and team-building tradition.

When the pasta party occurred on a Friday night prior to a high school football game, the runners were encouraged to attend only the first half of the game so they could get home to get eight hours of sleep. Some coaches might take a harder line about not doing anything prior to race day. As seriously as we know our sport needs to be approached, committed athletes are still high school kids. Within reason, I allowed them to enjoy as much of a full high school experience as possible.

I encouraged the runners to have their uniform, sweats, shoes, water bottles, towel, extra socks, dry clothes, and racing shoes laid out the night before. That way there was no panic in the morning just before leaving for the race.

Race Day

The schedule may vary depending on whether the race time is a weekday afternoon meet or a classic Saturday morning meet. Regardless, provide the runners with a detailed schedule for the day. (See **Appendix 4**.) Include bus departure times and expected arrival times at the meet for athletes who are self-transporting. For each race of the day, have a detailed warmup and cool-down schedule that details times, including bathroom breaks. Assign group captain(s) for each team to get the athletes warming up at the listed time, which is especially helpful when races might be scheduled too close together for coaches to manage all warmups or even get runners to the starting lines.

It is particularly important to get accurate split times and finishing places for everyone in each race. Injured runners, parents, assistant coaches, or runners who have already run can be assigned to record this information. Have them enter the data directly into a computer so the split sheet (see **Resources**) can be sent out immediately for runners and parents to study along with the season summary of all their times to date. (See **Resources** for samples.)

An important thing for the runners to do on race day, which helps with their confidence and positivity, is the exact same warmup and drill routine that they do each day at practice. This familiar routine is grounding and stabilizing. Once the warmup is completed, have them change into racing flats (if using), adjust uniforms, make sure bibs/timing chips are in place, and top off fluids before heading to the start line. I like to have them at the start in time to do several (four to six) stride outs to stay loose and burn off some of the nervous energy. Do not let them just stand around because they lose their warmup that way.

Upon finishing the race, my runners all practiced the "Nekota Rule." Years ago, there was a wonderful runner from our Orange County area named Kay Nekota. Most often, Kay would finish in first place, yet she would wait at the finish line and congratulate each and every runner—from all teams—who finished after her. It was a remarkable illustration of sportsmanship and camaraderie. My runners adopted this practice until all of our school runners finished. That way, they returned together as one team back to our tent area to begin the rest of their post-race routines.

CHAPTER 5:

THE MENTAL RACE

How to Have Confidence on Race Day

Helping athletes relax and stay focused before a meet is an important challenge to be met. In keeping with my theme so far, I encourage you to do your own research for articles, videos, and websites that can help instruct you and your runners. Having your runners share their own ideas with each other is especially helpful. Have a panel of veterans share their experiences, fears, mantras, and favorite mental gimmicks.

Some of my approaches and insights can hopefully serve as a springboard for you to develop your own approach to this important area of racing.

Former Olympian Lynn Jennings shared that her best races were ones in which she wanted to quit halfway through. Why? Because she was out on the edge, pushing herself physically, and having to fight herself mentally to keep pressing against that edge. The result was championship level performances. It is particularly important that runners know how much the mental race is a huge factor in determining their performance in the physical race.

The most important thing in the mental race is confidence. Confidence comes from positivity: positive self-image and positive thoughts about workouts, teammates, coaches, family, and friends. Everyone has doubts and negative thoughts. It is, however, what you choose to do with those thoughts that matters. I would never tell athletes that a workout was easy. The term *easy* was not used in our program. Runners need to be proud of themselves and gain confidence that comes from the knowledge of completing something difficult and doing it well, despite how hard it was.

All of us have a little, critical version of ourselves, sitting on our shoulders during races. This little self tells us we are going too fast. It challenges our sanity. It demands that we slow down. It ridicules us for thinking we can race at such a pace. The voice is negative and demeaning and critical. Now here is the key: Do not tell them to ignore that voice. Instead, have an answer ready. The secret is to respond with positive facts, such as, "I have done the workouts to be able to go this fast . . . I have trained for this goal . . . I have prepared for this challenge, for this race, for these competitors." Make sure your runners have an answer that emphasizes positive and fact-based responses to dismantle that negative voice.

It is essential to provide real tools, as well as reinforcing positivity. The goal-setting activity described next helps provide positive, factual reinforcement of the runners' realistic goals, based on their own actual workout results. They can race this fast because they have practiced for it and planned for it.

Goal Setting

The day before each race my teams met in a classroom setting to discuss the course and scout opponents, go over lineups, practice mental imagery, and complete goal-setting sheets (see **Appendix 6** for a sample). I used a PowerPoint presentation and/or a handout to provide visual information that helped the runners set realistically high goals for the race. I reviewed the results from the previous years' race, if applicable, to help them predict likely finish places, compare the course to previously run courses, and sometimes, even to provide details on predicting their ideal finish times, based on workouts and previous races.

Runners used the Goal Sheet to write down and commit to their goal time, place, pace, and what they specifically planned to do to execute this plan. Following the race—either the next day or at the next prerace meeting—athletes completed a self-evaluation of their race. All were required to include three things they did well and three things they wanted to improve for the next race.

This self-examination/documentation is particularly important and productive. Everyone needs to know where they currently stand, where they are going, and how to achieve and get there. When there is weakness, it is imperative to understand it. The more the runners know, the clearer and more confident they can be about the plan to improve.

The power of visualization is vital to success in running. My runners always did a mental race_prior to the actual race. Research has shown that a focused mental approach has statistically significant physical benefits. Visualizing a race in their mind can cause a runner to race faster. It is science! Teach the mental race technique prior to the first race of the season. Have the runners lie down or put their heads on a classroom desk. Tell them to relax and begin to visualize the race site and scene as you describe it. Take them through the race from start to finish in approximately three minutes. Emphasize positive visual cues. Here is a brief example:

"You are at the starting line, and you feel great. Your warmup was the best. You know you are prepared. You know you have a great race plan. The starting gun goes off, and you get a terrific start—not too fast . . . exactly right. You settle into a good spot and make that first turn. You are right where you want to be. As the race continues, you start to pick off runners who started too fast. You hit the first mile mark and check your split. You are on pace, and more importantly, you are feeling the best you have ever felt in the first mile."

The mental race goes on until the runner crosses the finish line in a great position and with a time under what he/she has planned. The athlete feels great.

The final tools for mental race preparation are called *mantras*. These are short phrases that the athlete can repeat over and over again to give themselves confidence, fight negativity, and have something to focus on when things inevitably get tough. Examples of mantras are, "I can do this," "I am prepared," or "I am strong."

CASE STUDY: ASHLEY LICATA

Overcoming Race Day Nerves to Become a Champion

Ashley Licata, recently graduated from the University of Utah where she was on the cross country and track and field teams following her career at Capistrano Valley High, was one of the hardest working, most dedicated runners I ever had the pleasure of coaching.

Her career with CVHS began with a remarkable freshman season culminating in a personal record of 17:34. As a sophomore, she improved that time a bit, and then in her junior year, she dropped her best to 17:07. Eventually, as a senior, she would run 17:04 and have accumulated seven times under 17:28. For these accomplishments, she was a multiple league and county first teamer. She advanced to four State Championships with our program. These records and recognitions brought her to the University of Utah.

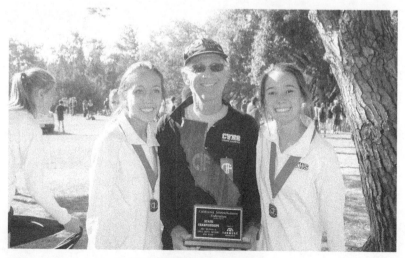

State with Mikaela and Ashley

Race days, however, were not easy for Ashley . . . until they were over. Ashley had worked hard and prepared well for her races, but her high expectations for her own performances caused race-day anxiety that was often difficult for her to cope with. Clearly, she did overcome it, but it took our support, positivity, and her immense intestinal fortitude to prevail. I helped her with visualization and race planning as described in the "Mental Race" chapter earlier. In particular, it was important for Ashley to remember who she was and what she had done. She had done the workouts at a remarkably high level. With each passing race, she had evidence of how good she was and how her work had paid off.

I would remind her of the evidence of her excellence as a way of boosting her confidence. Each great workout and each wonderful race finish were testimonies of her greatness. As her high school career moved forward, these bouts of self-doubt and anxiety lessened as she learned to focus on who she was—a champion many times over.

CHAPTER 6:

PREPARING AND REPAIRING

Fuel, Fluids, and Injuries

I n this chapter, I will touch quickly on subjects that are important to the overall health and safety of your runners. You can certainly find lots of detailed and comprehensive information on these topics online and in other publications. My purpose here is to raise your awareness of the need to educate yourself, your athletes, and parents in these areas.

Hydration

Most of us are generally aware of the need to stay hydrated. As a runner there are two particularly important reasons. First, the health and safety of the athlete depends on proper hydration. The second reason is performance correlations. Poor hydration can lead to dire consequences, especially in the heat. Performance suffers with as a little as a 2 percent loss of fluid balance. When a runner is not sufficiently hydrated, the blood, which is primarily liquid, thickens.

Therefore, it becomes harder for the heart to pump oxygen out to muscles during exercise.

How do you get your runners to hydrate appropriately? You must harp on it constantly. I talked about it every day. I reminded runners to drink several times during practice. You could even require them to show you their fluid supply as part of their check-in for practice at roll call. No fluids, no practice!

How much fluids are needed? There are a wide variety of formulas for proper hydration. In my experience, an athlete needs at least sixteen ounces upon waking, another sixteen ounces during the day prior to the afternoon practices, and yet another sixteen ounces during practice. Immediately following practice, they should have enough fluid to replace fluids lost during practice. This leads to the most important test of hydration: the urine test.

Urine should be relatively clear, not yellow. The darker it is, the less hydrated the runner is. Absolutely clear urine may indicate too much hydration, which can also be a problem. The athlete may be flushing out too many good nutrients by overhydration. You may have heard of this formula: a minimum of one-third of body weight in fluids as a base point and then enough fluid to replace what is lost during exercise (checked by the urine test).

In addition to the visual urine test, weighing oneself before and after a workout is also a particularly good measurement of how much fluid was lost. Within an hour or so of finishing practice, a runner should have hydrated enough to be near their pre-workout weight. An unfortunate downside with female runners and weighing is the attention it may bring to possible body image issues they may have. There is no easy solution to that issue. Speak directly by acknowledging the attention brought to weight but emphasize the importance of knowledge about hydration. They should not weigh every day or every workout. Have them weigh once or twice a week to see what normal weight loss might be after a workout, and then they should have enough information available to account for that loss of weight.

As to what to drink, it is important to emphasize that drinking only water may not be sufficient to account for the loss of minerals, including sodium and potassium. Certainly, a good diet that includes good sources of sodium and potassium can help a lot. However, using a sports drink along with water or mixed with water is necessary. Articles you may read or refer your runners to will point out trying to avoid any drinks with too much sugar. If you study comparisons of the major sports drinks, you will not find significant differences between drinks. Stress finding the drink they like and will use.

In addition to the general recommendations I made about hydration, here is some more specific information: Many authors suggest avoiding fluid consumption in the twenty minutes prior to a workout. This keeps the stomach from feeling too full. Most experts suggest six to eight ounces every fifteen to twenty minutes during a workout. An ounce is generally a swallow. A trick I discovered through some research indicates that if a swallow of liquid is put in your mouth, swished around, and spit out, it actually tricks the body into thinking it received more hydration than was actually the case. This can help maintain proper hydration during workouts without that bloated feeling.

Nutrition

There is certainly an abundance of articles and books on the subject of nutrition for runners. I will highlight some key considerations when dealing with this topic.

There will be some constraints when working with your athletes and families. Each family has its own nutritional habits, budgets, and cultural customs/traditions regarding food. There may be some resistance to overcoming these as you attempt to get your runners to eat an ideal nutritional plan. Do what is possible to educate your families by sending home articles and brief emails to educate and inform. Try to keep it simple, practical, and brief.

Getting the athletes to focus on and be attentive to fuel intake can be exceedingly difficult. Some coaches use food diaries specific for running. Runners can also do a one-time food analysis for seven days. This helps identify balances, intake, habits—both good and bad—and where improvement is indicated. This creates some self-awareness. Ultimately, the implementation responsibilities for healthy nutrition remain with each athlete and their families.

First and foremost, stress the importance of proper nutrition to your athletes and families. I used the image of an engine and fuel. The body is the engine that runs the races for each athlete. Just like no one would start a race in a car without adequate gas, no one should imagine that the body will function in workouts and races without the proper type and amount of food. There may be lots of excuses from athletes about why they cannot fuel appropriately—that they do not like certain foods is the predominant excuse. Be vigilant in using the fuel/car imagery. A car runs out of gas if it is not fueled, and so will a runner!

The second point regarding nutrition is that most endurance athletes are looking for a balance of 60 percent carbohydrates, 25 percent protein, and 15 percent fat, give or take 5 percent. Distance runners, and females in particular, have to be careful about having too little fat in their diet. Too little fat can lead to an increase in injuries. Additionally, fat is a source of energy. Studies show that the existence of sufficient fat stores in the body prolongs the time when the body taps into the carbohydrate stores, which sustains the length of time the runner can run. This is a good thing for a distance runner.

RED-S (Formerly known as THE FEMALE TRIAD)

Relative Energy Deficiency in Sport (RED-S) is a condition that implies inadequate energy intake relative to the energy needed as an athlete. In females it is characterized by disordered eating, amenorrhea/oligomenorrhoea (absence of or irregular menstrual cycles), and decreased bone mineral density. It leads to, at a minimum, decreased performance and increased injuries. This is a serious illness with life-long health consequences that can even be fatal. It is mainly found in female athletes in sports that emphasize leanness and low body weight, but sometimes, symptoms can be found in men, as well.

RED-S is not caused by exercise or by being an athlete. It can begin with the pressure to lose weight. Dieting often leads to energy drain, and this, combined with the demands for the energy needed as a distance athlete, can lead to a dangerous spiral of bodily reactions. The body could stop the reproductive system in response to extreme weight loss and high physical demands. In women, this can lead to a lack in production of hormones necessary for bone formation. Osteoporosis may result, which means old bones are found in young women.

What can a coach do about RED-S? Educate yourself and share that information with your runners and families. Deemphasize weight goals and focus on overall health. Offer plenty of information about healthy eating habits. Provide appropriate role models to assist in the runners' internalization of what a healthy runner looks like in terms of body image.

Positive Body Images and the Real World of Growth

Early in my career, I had two female stars who grew up quickly over a summer. As freshmen and sophomores with underdeveloped, child-like bodies, they ran extremely fast. As they matured and their bodies changed, their performance as juniors became dramatically slower. Their parents questioned me about how I was coaching them and basically wanted to blame me for their decline in performance. I thought to myself, (but did not say to them), "Are they not seeing the changes in the girls' bodies?" Mother Nature has her own plan.

Discussing this with female runners and their parents is certainly not an easy task, but I think it's a necessary one. I suggest trying to find an article you can share on the subject of natural development, weight gain, and growth in young females. Perhaps include it among other educational materials about nutrition and positive self-image. If you are a male coach and have a female assistant coach, this might be a task for her to take on.

Iron and Ferritin

Over the years, I have had several girls, including championship and university-bound runners, who have suffered from a lack of iron binding. This is *not* just a lack of iron itself. It is a failure of the iron to bind to hemoglobin, which is needed so that oxygen transfers to the lungs and muscles, enabling the athlete to run faster and farther. An indicator of this problem can present as a lack of energy near the end of workouts or races and, sometimes, increased sweat rates. Often, outstanding runners would end up dropping out of races or workouts with sheer fatigue, unexplained by anything else.

As part of the yearly physical required for school clearance to participate in sports, I recommend a ferritin binding test. This is a test of how the iron in the body is binding. It can save an athlete a lot of grief if the problem is diagnosed early.

Have the athletes make sure the doctor is clear that this patient is an endurance runner. The normal number from a test may be around twenty-five or thirty, but a runner needs it to be more like fifty to sixty, or higher. I spoke with Olympian Shalane Flannagan at NXN a few years ago. As a female marathoner, she wanted her number to be close to a one hundred! The breakdown and rebuilding of muscle tissue as a result of training and racing requires more iron than the average person. Young females have the additional need for iron for their menstrual cycles, which can be particularly depleted by exercise.

Early identification of this problem is crucial because it can take *months* of diet and supplements to correct, possibly destroying an entire season. I am not a doctor, but my experiences with athletes and families, along with my research, do indicate a number of solutions that should be discussed with a professional. These include various forms of iron supplements, including liquid iron. All the supplements require professional dietary monitoring to make certain the iron is absorbed and retained. Some foods negate the effects sought by the supplement. Known iron inhibitors include calcium, tea, coffee, and eggs. Some forms of liquid iron must be taken *without* food. Be careful and always consult with a professional.

CASE STUDY: ALYSSA BAUTISTA
Swimming to UCLA Through Iron-Deficient Waters

Alyssa was a swimmer and wanted to join the cross-country team at Capistrano Valley High to help her get in better shape for the swim season. She was a very accomplished local swimmer and had no thoughts of a career as a top high school distance runner. How quickly things changed!

In her first two high school races, she and her teammate, Haley Herberg, thoroughly dominated their competition with Alyssa running a stunning 17:48 in only her second race ever. She had a couple of injuries that slowed her development as a freshman, but her stunning career was on its way. Her success at cross country and her love of running and for the team around her caused her to move on from swimming and focus just on her career as a distance runner.

As a sophomore, she ran in the high seventeens often, and then as a junior, exploded with a 16:57 personal best. During the ensuing track and field seasons, she became an 800-meter specialist, winning multiple league championships and qualifying for CIF SS Finals several times. She eventually had a best time of 2:12.63. Her senior season of cross country led to her finishing her career with five sub-17:10 runs and a fourth-place finish at the State Cross Country Championships. She went on to qualify for the Footlocker National Individual Championships race, becoming an official high school All-American. Her thoughts of swimming were far behind her as she was offered a scholarship to run for University of California at Los Angeles (UCLA).

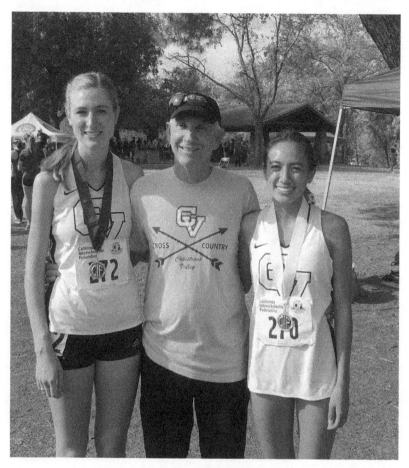

Coach with Haley and Alyssa

Alyssa battled with iron-binding issues as discussed in Chapter 11. She and her family consulted with doctors and developed the appropriate diet and supplement plan to help overcome the iron-binding deficiency, which had caused her to not be able to finish workouts and race below her capabilities.

This condition can take months to correct, and if not dealt with aggressively and early, can cause an athlete to lose an entire season. To her credit, Alyssa, with the support of her wonderful family, fought through the challenges and ended up a Bruin as a result.

Coping with the Elements

As a native Southern Californian who has lived and coached my entire life in this area, I know I have a laughably inadequate experience with weather extremes compared to most coaches and runners in the country, though we do have some extreme heat here. Nevertheless, I will relay a bit of information and one particular tip that I hope you find useful.

Heat

Heat is particularly dangerous for runners given the impact it has on fluid loss and hydration. There are many charts and tables to help calculate heat and humidity and their impact on running. Your state or regional athletic governance may also send out warnings, alerts, and charts to help calculate the impact and risk of exercise under heat and humidity extremes. The heat extremes in Southern California during the afternoons in summertime and early fall can mean temperatures over one hundred degrees Fahrenheit. Aside from the obvious emphasis on hydration, there are several things I suggest to modify workouts without eliminating them altogether:

- Shorten workouts by time or distance.
- Divide up workouts into smaller parts with hydration breaks in-between.
- Keep workouts on campus, in front of the coaches for constant supervision.
- Run inside the air-conditioned school building.
- Shift to pool workouts.
- Move workouts to the morning (though, can be a logistical problem with class schedules).

It is important to safely develop a positive mindset for athletes and parents regarding working out and racing in the heat. When runners have successfully coped with heat in workouts that you have designed with safety in mind, they will be more confident on race day.

Bronte Shirts

"Bronte Shirts" is a tool I developed in conjunction with a star athlete, her mom, and inspiration from marathoners Meb Keflezighi and Deena Kastor, who at the 2004 Athens Olympics, used this type of tool. Bronte was my star runner and eventually became the top runner at UCLA. She was strong, dedicated, rarely injured, and extremely fast but struggled in extreme heat. Something in her system did not handle heat well. Even though she hydrated properly, she became very flush and her performance suffered in heat. Prior to the League Finals race during her senior year, she was a favorite to win but genuinely concerned because the forecast for race time was for the mid- to high-90s.

I remembered that for the 2004 Olympic marathon in Athens, USA marathoners were provided with a unique experimental vest/jacket to wear during warmup. It contained ice or cold water in various pockets to keep the runners' core temperatures down in an effort to delay the onset of sweat until the last minute, thus prolonging dehydration. Of course, Meb earned the silver medal and Deena, the bronze. They attributed this invention for their ability to cope with the extreme heat and humidity. I spoke with Bronte about the jacket/vest idea the week before the race. She and her mom then took several t-shirts, soaked them in water, and put them in the freezer overnight. When she arrived at the race, she pulled several frozen shirts out of an ice chest and wore them while awaiting the race and during her warmup. She completely dominated the race and said she "never felt better during the heat." So, the Bronte Shirt was born. I have taught this trick to athletes and parents ever since. It has had a significant impact on the ability of my runners to perform better than most in severe heat.

CASE STUDY: BRONTE GOLICK
From Martial Arts to Bronte Shirts to Top UCLA Runner

In the summer of 2007, Bronte came to our first summer practices for cross country with some reluctance. She was, after all, not a runner. She was into martial arts. But Bronte had a neighbor on the Capistrano Valley High cross-country team. This young lady said that cross country was a way to get out of regular PE class and that it was a fun group of girls with a nice guy for a coach.

As that coach, I can report that she was an average runner early that summer. She routinely ran in the nine-minute range on the distance runs. She did have a particularly good form, however, and I began to encourage her to pull away from the group of friends she was running with and challenge herself more. At her first race, she ran just under twenty-two minutes on a hilly course. By the end of her freshman year, she was running just under nineteen minutes and beginning to show the promise of things to come.

During her sophomore year, she became a varsity runner and advanced to a 17:58, her best time. She demonstrated an incredible work ethic and a fierce competitive nature, both of which would carry her through her career.

During her junior year, Bronte really broke out with a best time of 17:40—at that time, a school record. In her senior year, she ran a personal best of 17:29, won the League Championship and advanced to CIF SS finals for the second straight year, just missing a second State Meet qualification by a second.

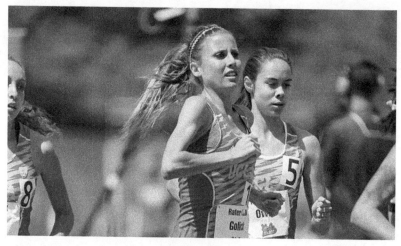

Bronte Golick

It was during the Sea View League Championships that year that the Bronte Shirt came into play as described earlier. She went on to earn a scholarship to UCLA, where she eventually became their top distance runner.

Bronte's case demonstrates two things. First, even reluctant participants can find a place on a team. With hard work and focus, they can become stars. Secondly, though adversity may appear to limit a runner's possible achievements, ingenuity and perseverance can lead to championships.

Cold

So again, I thank the majority of the country for not laughing too hard here as the native Southern Californian discusses running in the cold. Much can be found in online research that is helpful. In many ways, it is much simpler than dealing with the heat.

Cover up! Tights or sweatpants over tights is a good start to keeping the legs warm. Layer the upper body. The heart pumps blood to the brain and big muscles first. The far extremities, such as fingers and toes, need to be well covered. Wear gloves and a hat. The head releases a lot of heat that can be channeled back into the body with a good hat or knit cap. I believe in the twenty-degree rule. Your body will think it is twenty degrees warmer after fifteen to twenty minutes of running. Layering helps to start out warm, and then maybe shed a layer or two as the runner warms up, depending on the temperature.

Injuries and Injury Prevention

In keeping with my approach throughout this book, I intend this to be a brief discussion of some things you may want to explore, research, and implement in much more detail. There is a lot of information available out there.

Trainers

Some schools have an onsite trainer assigned to work with athletic teams throughout the year. It is important to establish a good relationship with this person. Introduce yourself and invite them to come by your practice site to introduce themselves to the runners.

Make sure your athletes know where the trainer's office is located. Ask the trainer to bring ice and water to practice on a regular basis. A note of caution: If you have some less than dedicated runners, they may decide when they want to be injured and want to spend more time with the trainer than at practice. Set up some guidelines and procedures about when and how runners are allowed to go to the trainer and for what purposes. Work with the trainer to set up these protocols, and make the expectations known in writing so that you can hold the athletes accountable.

Education/Information

Though old-school in delivery, I found it helpful to have a set of paper files with hard copy articles about specific injuries and how to diagnose and treat them. Many articles were from popular running magazines. If a runner had a particular concern, I could instantly hand her a page or two and ask her to read and discuss it with me. Putting together links to such articles on your website is also encouraged. The most common injuries are: runner's knee, iliotibial band syndrome, shin splints, Achilles and arch injuries, hamstring injuries, and gluteus (butt) pain.

Pain vs. Strain

The most difficult part of injuries with athletes is helping them to distinguish the difference between the pain that is injury-related and the pain from soreness as a result of hard work. Training at a high championship level is very demanding and involves lots of pain in the non-injury sense of the word. If runners are not tired and sore after a workout, they are not working hard enough.

No distance runner doing their best to improve is likely to feel fine. Something is always tired, sore, fatigued, or even painful. Helping runners learn the difference between pain that is injury-related versus soreness from hard work is a delicate balance. There are no easy ways to make this determination. However, here are some things to try:

- Ask, "Does the hurt area warm up and feel better or get worse as practice moves on?" If it worsens, it is more likely an injury. If it is better, it may be a sore muscle but something to keep an eye on.
- Ask, "Are you limping or favoring something?" If so, it is definitely an injury situation that needs to be cared for professionally.
- Ask, "What in the workout makes it better or worse?" This may give an answer as to what is wrong.

The bottom line is this: If you have a trainer you trust, send the athlete to the trainer immediately. Quick interventions cover you in a practical, liability sense and may provide more insights about the issue.

Tools

If your school or booster budget permits, here are some items to purchase for your team to help with injury prevention and rehabilitation:

- Foam rollers: have athletes routinely use rollers, especially those with IT band, glute, hamstring, and quad soreness.
- Stick massagers: there are various types that have rollers or raised surfaces; they are usually used with two hands on tight and sore areas.
- Power massagers: these are pricier, but if you get a couple of them, they can work wonders.
- Elastic straps: these are excellent for hip strengthening. Search online for how to use them, but basically, you sidestep with the strap around your lower legs.

Cross Training

There is absolutely no substitute for running when you want to be a runner. I have done much cross training in my own running/triathlon career and found it to be useful and productive.

My experience and understanding have caused me to believe cross training should be used as a supplement and not a replacement for healthy runners. Certainly, for injured athletes or rehabilitation situations, cross training takes on a more primary focus. Here are some cross training options:

- Pool running: this is an excellent option for injured runners.
- Elliptical trainer: this is not quite the running motion but comes close, depending on the variety of equipment. It is impact free.
- Stationary bike: negates the pounding but simulates running workouts fairly easily.

- Regular road or mountain bike: the problem with this is that unless it's all flat, half of the time, you are coasting.
- Swimming: this is good for aerobic development but not very muscle specific for runners

Cross-Country Weight Training

Ideally, weight training should take place two to three times a week, starting in the summer and continuing into early October, then two times a week during mid and late October, dropping to once a week during championship time. The goal is not to build bulk and definition but rather to strengthen specific running muscles, as well as prevent injury. Consistent weight training, along with good core work, will improve race times ten to twenty seconds per mile.

Warmup First

Prior to lifting weights, a warmup is necessary. Options include at least ten minutes of running, cycling, stair climbing, or elliptical. Many runners find that doing weight work after a run ensures that muscles are loose and extends the time their heart rate is raised. This burns additional calories, too.

Exercises to Include

Generally, design workouts that strengthen the *upper body*, so the arm swing and arm drive will be forceful and consistent throughout workouts and races. Exercises to help the *lower body* provide enough support to the bones and ligaments and allow for fast running on all terrains. Be very conscious of the *core* area. Runners have to keep the abdominal and back muscles strong. Many running-related injuries are due to a weak core that results in imbalances and leads to injuries and poor performance.

Number of Repetitions

When you begin, do two sets of twelve to fifteen repetitions of each exercise. After a month, add a third set. Do eight to ten exercises in one session. Another *great* way to do these is in a circuit, completing one exercise and then moving on to the next quickly to complete three sets.

Amount of Weight

There are many formulas, but simply use the weight that will allow for completion of the sets and repetitions suggested. **What are some specific weight exercises for runners?** This can vary depending on the equipment you have access to. The list below will not be a comprehensive one but generally shows the types of exercises that emphasize important areas for runners.

UPPER BODY—Common Exercises May Include:

- Bench press: lie on back and press weights straight up to ceiling.
- Chest press: use a slanted bench or sit up, hold the weights straight overhead, and pull down.
- Arm curls: stand or sit with weights in hand and pull toward chest.
- Lat pull down: on a machine, facing weights, pull in front and behind the neck.
- Triceps curl: hold a dumbbell behind head/neck, raise above head by straightening the arms.
- Bent row: kneel over bench, back flat, raise one dumbbell to shoulder, keeping arm straight.
- Arm swing: hold a weight in each arm, swing arms in running motion for two minutes.

- Triceps pull down: facing a machine with a weight at chest, pull down to waist with arms.

LOWER BODY–Common Exercises May Include:

- Leg extensions: seated on a machine, lift legs by straightening, works quadriceps.
- Leg curls: lying on stomach, bring heels to buttocks, works hamstrings.
- Quarter squats: with bar or dumbbell, using both legs at same time.
- Lunge: with a bar or dumbbell, go lower so knee almost to ground.
- Leg press: place legs on platform provided and extend legs to straight
- Toe or calf raises: on machine while holding dumbbells.

CORE WORK–Try to Do One hundred Pushups and 200 Sit-ups a Day.

(See **Appendix 7**) for a sample workout.

Injuries and Grades

If you provide grades for a report card, and if you are inclined to actually make runners accountable and not give all As, accounting for injuries is a challenge. A note from the trainer or a doctor may be required. While not able to run, injured athletes need to be doing something of a cross training nature or help document workout times and do paperwork to keep their grades up. In my program, runners could not get an A unless they actually raced. Injured runners could come close to an A by helping to take times and counting places at each mile and at the finish, along with data entry and record keeping of race results. See (**Appendix 8)** for a sample grading policy.

CHAPTER 7:

TRICKS OF THE TRADE

Breathing, Form, and Hills

I t is important to do as much teaching as possible in the early part of the summer so that the athletes and parents understand what the running goals are and how they will be accomplished. It is also important not to give the athletes too much to think about at one time, so I spread those instructional moments out over the first five weeks of training in small five- or ten-minute increments. In addition to the topics in the following chapter, I sent home a brief explanation of the workout system (see **Appendix 1**) and definitions of the types of workouts to parents and athletes.

Here are some of the topics to cover early in the summer:

Tying Your Shoes

I need to give the great University of California at Los Angeles (UCLA) basketball coach, John Wooden, credit for this idea and my adaptation of it. At the first practice of a season composed of future All Americans and Hall of Famers, Wooden spent a significant amount of time teaching them something basic: how to tie their shoes.

He explained why it was important and had them practice doing it, over and over again! For runners, the only piece of equipment that really matters in their performance is their shoes. The shoes need to be tied properly, not be too tight, and not be too loose, to reduce blisters. More importantly, the shoes need to be re-tied at least once after putting them on, before the actual workout starts but after warming up, as the foot, the shoe, and the laces all change dimension with heat and blood flow. I demonstrated how much more lace I had left to tie the laces tight after my initial morning lace-up. Just like a biker's hard shoe in a cleat directs the energy for the pedaling, a solid platform in the form of a shoe concentrates the energy for a runner. Any movement inside the shoe that does not help the foot move directly forward is a waste of energy. Over a three mile/5k race, this could result in a minute or more of wasted time. Remind the athletes for several days about proper shoe tying and then, eventually, less frequently as they adopt it as a regular habit.

Form

In the first day or two of practice, go over proper running form. Reinforce it several times over the first few weeks until habits are ingrained. Start by instructing the runners to stand tall, imagining a balloon pulling up from the top of the head. Next, have them be conscious of pulling in a bit on the belly button to help position the hips underneath them. They should relax the shoulders and let the arms hang loosely. Have them raise their hands to a running position without raising the shoulders. Tell them to lift the hands up to a bit above waist level, keeping the shoulders still. The hands need to be relaxed—no fists or tension. The arm swing should keep the elbows near the body, and the hands should not cross over the midline of the body. Crossover causes the shoulders, and then the body, to move from side to side rather than forward and is very inefficient. Once an athlete is running, foot placement should be midfoot forward—not on the heels and not on the toes.

Breathing, Rhythmic Breathing, and Side Stitches

Teach runners to breathe from the diaphragm (or stomach) and not the upper chest. One way I found to do this was to have them put one hand on their chest and one hand on their stomach. Ask them to see if they can tell where more of the movement is originating from. The stomach should be driving the breath, not the chest. The chest is too shallow and not enough oxygen is circulated.

Remind runners to be aware of the pattern of their own breathing. Here, I refer you to the book *Running on Air* by Budd Coates and Claire Kowalchik of *Runner's World* magazine. The book describes how to use rhythmic breathing to maximize oxygen intake, which also minimizes side stitches. Research suggests that the source of the side stitch is constant inhalation on the same side. Because the diaphragm is a muscle, it becomes stressed or fatigued by the impact of the foot strike when a runner is breathing in. By alternating the side or leg of the inhale, the impact on one side is cut in half, thus reducing, or eliminating, side stitches. I have run over 70,000 miles in my running career and *never* had a side stitch. I have come to realize that I just naturally fell into this rhythmic breathing pattern. So, breathe in on the left foot, step with the right, step with the left, next, breathe in on the right foot, step with the left, step with the right, and finally, breathe in on the left foot.

Stride Frequency, Stride Length, and Foot Strike

Usually, on the second day of practice, I asked the runners to count how many times their right foot hit the ground in sixty seconds of moderately paced running. Experts suggest that the ideal number should be ninety (180 if counting both feet). Given the slightly unscientific nature of this test, a range of eighty-eight to ninety-two is considered good. Those who fall well below (low eighties) are striding too long and/or spending too much time in the air between foot strikes. This is inefficient and does not propel the runner forward with the least amount of effort, which is the goal. Those whose number is much higher (mid to high nineties) are taking too many steps and/or have too short a stride length. They are using too much energy for too little pay off in moving forward.

Most of the time, the over-strider is a taller runner, and the under-strider is shorter. This may be a function of the runners' leg lengths. It is also likely that some muscle weaknesses prevent the short strider from lifting the leg up and out. I found that out of fifty girls, more than forty would be in the normal range, four to six were under the goal number (striding less frequently than was ideal), and two to three were over the goal number (striding more frequently than was ideal).

You may find articles from various sources to help you correct these inefficiencies. It takes a lot of conscious work on the part of the runner to alter what may be several years of muscle memory, so I caution you to be patient and persistent. In the case of the long, slow strider, instruct them to consciously practice a slightly quicker turnover or stride frequency. If the long, slow strider is also a heel striker (which is hard on the knees and back), encourage them to land more on the midfoot to mid forefront of the foot, which may increase the turnover rate slightly. For the short quick strider, help them be conscious of extending the foot and leg farther out in front of them without heel striking. It may be that the hip flexor and related muscles and tendons are weak, so having the runners do more lunge-type exercises is important.

Hill Technique

I divide hill form discussions into two obvious parts: uphill and downhill.

Uphill technique has several parts. Do not bend over too far or lean too far into a hill. It causes bad form and limits proper breathing. Try to stay upright. An aggressive arm swing is essential. The steeper the hill, the more exaggerated the arm swing needs to be. It helps lift the legs so that the runner does not end up with short, choppy steps, which result in loss of power and speed. Finally, cresting is especially important. That is, do not relax the effort when reaching the top of a hill. Take two to four quick strides to reestablish a normal stride length as was used approaching the top, otherwise, the tendency is to be in the shorter stride mode that uphill running often creates.

Downhill technique also has several parts. It is important to stay balanced. This is achieved in several ways. Land midfoot instead of using the braking motion that heel striking brings. Most importantly, substantially increase turnover or stride frequency. This keeps the runner's feet on the ground more often increasing the sense of stability and balance. Finally, some experts suggest making an adjustment with the arms. Moving them a bit wider for balance is the simplest and least energetic strategy.

Hill Attitude and Approach

Many studies have demonstrated that trying too hard while running uphill is ultimately more costly in terms of energy use and cannot be covered by the ease of the downhill. It is best to keep a steady effort with good technique. Make use of the cresting technique and run downhill with an aggressive attitude. My experience with runners at the famously hilly Mt. Sac course is that really aggressive downhill running is a key to winning races on hilly courses.

Pool Running

You can find several articles and books on the various ways to use a pool for cross training, injury prevention, and rehabilitation. I will briefly describe how I made use of it. Hopefully, you have a pool at your school. Establish a relationship with the aquatics people to allow for pool access.

I did not use swim-type workouts; although, they certainly can be worthwhile for aerobic development. Instead, my runners practiced the basic running motion in the pool. Waist belts of some sort may be used during this exercise. They keep the runner upright and in better form. However, the effort is harder without the belt. The core strengthening that results from keeping upright without the belt has many benefits. Vary pool workouts. Do easy pool running with various fast and slow combinations just to change the motion and keep the interest level way up.

CHAPTER 8:

A CHAMPIONSHIP MINDSET

Deciding to Be the Best

want to tell you a story. In the summer of 2012, I invited about twenty of our projected top runners to our special training camp in Mammoth Lakes, located in the Sierra Nevada Mountains in California. For many years we had been a "good" program in Southern California, making the CIF prelims most years and frequently the CIF finals. We usually finished in the top six to ten range in the highly competitive Orange County Championship races. Still, we were not a "great" program. I studied and read, talked with other coaches, and attended seminars, but we were still missing something to get to the next level.

As I was preparing for the education seminars, I knew I'd have two periods in the day at camp, between workouts and meals. I ran (no pun intended) across an ad for a video called, "Run with Your Body, Race with Your Mind" by Dr. Stan Beecham. It looked interesting. I sent away for it, and upon receiving it, threw it in my backpack, and hauled it up to Mammoth. Good teaching methodology would suggest previewing a DVD ahead of time to make sure it is relevant and appropriate for the learners. I did not do that! Instead, I apologized to the girls ahead of time, put on the DVD, and watched. My life and those of my teams changed because of the next few minutes watching the video.

In it, Dr. Beecham addressed a room of runners and asked them what their goals were. Many responded with a race time like 17:59 or 15:59. He asked why they chose that particular number, and they, of course, responded that they wanted to break eighteen or sixteen minutes. He then asked, "Why not 17:30 or 15:30?" Often, there was no answer. Dr Beecham went on to challenge the runners to examine why they were not reaching for higher, faster times. What would happen if they tried for the faster goal and failed? Would they get kicked off the team? Get a bad grade? No, of course not. What might happen was, if they trained properly and focused their mind correctly, they might actually achieve that faster time. *But they would never get there if they didn't try*!

When the DVD was over, it became so clear to me what was holding my runners back. I, their coach, was holding them back by not setting our team and individual goals higher, and, in turn, not setting up the workouts to achieve those higher goals. I had said I wanted us to finish among the top three in our league (one of toughest in the nation), so that we could go to the CIF playoffs. Why wasn't I saying that I wanted us to win our league? I had always explained that we wanted to be in the top eight in Orange County (one of the most competitive races short of a California State Meet). Why did I not say we wanted to be the County Champions?

Why was I (not) doing this? I was afraid to "fail." I was afraid to set my teams up for disappointment. Was I really going to get "fired" for being sixth and not first in Orange County? Were the athletes going to be more disappointed at not being first than at being seventh? My athletes and I vowed then and there, as a team, to never settle for trying to be less than the best. We understood we might not reach number one, but at least we wanted to try by pushing our own limits.

Two months later, we would have placed first at the Orange County Championships if not for a key injury during the race, and a month after that, we qualified for the California State Meet in Division One (large schools) for the first time. We would go on to win the Orange County title in 2013 and 2014, and we finished in the top three there for seven years in a row. We also qualified for the State Meet for six straight years, finishing second to Nike Cross Nationals (NXN) Top 10, Saugus High, and ranking as high as eighth nationally. We expected to win. We expected to be first, and we planned our workouts to get to the State Meet and beyond. Why not be *first*? *Thank you to Dr. Beecham!*

I have created a sample of a season-long goal-setting sheet (see **Resources**). I went over it with my top runners early in the summer at our special summer training camp in Mammoth. In it, I planned backward from our ultimate goal, the California State Meet. I listed the times the athletes needed to be running at each meet to progress toward that goal of making the State Meet. I researched the finishing times at the last State Meet as a starting point. Each week before the State Meet, I calculated what would need to be run on those specific courses and at those specific races. I continued listing the times to be run at each race all the way back to the first meet of the season. All workouts in my system (see the "Training" chapter) needed to be built to enable the runners to run those times at those meets.

CHAPTER 9:

STARTING A HIGH SCHOOL PROGRAM

Who are the Runners?

L et me remind the reader that I was a California-based pub-
lic-school coach. California has rules regarding the conduct of in-
terscholastic sports, and for cross country in particular, that may
differ from other areas of the country. I will attempt to be general in
my discussion of rules, but I remind you from the outset, especially
if you are a newcomer to coaching, to make sure that you are clear
about what your school, district, region, and state authorities allow
you to do and not do. For some jurisdictions even the word "recruiting" may be viewed as "a violation" of the rules. At a public school
in California, I basically had to coach the athletes who came to the
school site based on the school attendance boundaries. I absolutely
could never reach out to athletes at other schools to try to lure them to
my school. I am using the term "recruiting" here to refer to encourag-

ing participation on your team by those already at your school or who will be legally coming to your school.

If you are a newcomer to coaching, get the roster from the last season of cross country and/or from the most recent spring track and field team. Contact all of those athletes. Introduce yourself and schedule a meeting with them. Be prepared to inspire them to come out for your sport. Suggestions for a "Newcomers Meeting" agenda will come later. Speaking of the track and field team, aside from the distance-running athletes, try to encourage everyone to try cross country in the summer and fall. You can enlist your veteran cross country and track and field distance runners to help with this. Hold a meeting with them all at a track and field practice or invite them to your campus-wide recruitment meeting. Depending on the sport season, you may find some takers, specifically from the soccer team. In my area at Dana Hills High School, legendary and nationally recognized coach, Tim Butler, was a Physical Education teacher who held tryout runs early in the semester to help identify possible runners for his cross-country team.

In California, the rules regarding contact with incoming freshmen were extremely specific. Be clear about the rules for contacting incoming freshmen in your state. In California, we cannot have direct contact with them, one-on one, until they have graduated from middle school and are out of school for the summer. This creates quite a challenge. The procedure at Capistrano Valley High School (CVHS) started with the athletic director (AD) taking flyers to the middle school for distribution in the spring. If it is similar for you, make sure you have your AD well-stocked with handouts and contact information well in advance. CVHS school also holds an Eighth Grade Expo early in the spring to promote all academic and extracurricular activities, sports, and clubs so that the incoming students and parents can see what is available at the school. If your school has such an event, have a table set up with flyers, previous trophies, pictures, and interest signup sheets. It is helpful to have veteran athletes available to meet with prospective runners since many recent arrivals to your program may still be in touch with and know some of these newcomers.

When your school has finished registering students for fall classes, ask for the roster of those who have signed up for cross country (assuming it is a class) and make sure incoming freshmen are included. Get home addresses, emails, parent names, phone numbers, etc. Create a group email so that you can begin contacting veterans and newcomers alike regarding upcoming meetings and summer training.

Contact all newcomers, whether freshman or not, and invite them to a Newcomers Meeting at or near the end of the semester. Again, check on the rules in your area for the timing. I have found the Newcomers Meeting to be an important and exciting opportunity to welcome the athletes and their parents. Have them meet team captains and Booster Club leaders as well as other parents.

Display trophies, plaques, team photos, uniforms, and other swag. Captains and assistant coaches should help with greeting and checking in the athletes and parents. This can be a time to either collect or pass out any paperwork you may require. Captains working with the Booster parents at our Newcomers Meetings typically offered a small gift of a sports drink and an energy bar with a team color ribbon on it, welcoming everyone to the program. During check-in, make sure you have a way to verify all of the contact information; be especially prepared to gather it from those not on your list previously. Some may have heard of the meeting and wanted to come and check it out at the last minute.

I began the meeting with a greeting as the head coach and then introduced assistant coaches, captains, and parent leaders who were present. Next, I presented a PowerPoint presentation that was an overview of the program with expectations and goals. It is a good idea to anticipate as many questions as possible by providing written materials, such as summer workout schedules, tips on how to prepare for upcoming practices, information on meets and pasta parties, and contact information for Booster leaders and coaches.

Here is a brief outline of topics to cover at the Newcomers Meeting:

- What is cross country? Discuss distances, league and section playoffs, and invitationals.
- How is the team constructed? Varsity, junior varsity (JV), sophomores, and freshman.
- How do you get on the team? Are there tryouts? Outline the minimum number of miles or practices.
- How do you prepare for summer practices? Discuss shoes, fluids, fuel, and watches.
- Explain registration, school paperwork requirements, including physicals, clearances, insurance info, and waivers.
- Stress the "family" and community aspect of the team, parents, and coaches.
- Go over the summer schedule and preview the fall schedule.
- Give some detail as to how the summer training works regarding attendance and miles, practice locations, and start and end times (See **Resources**).
- Cover the basics of periodization and types of workouts, which could include cross training.
- Highlight special summer camps you will offer and how runners become eligible to attend.
- If your team meets as an actual class in the fall as part of the school day, explain how that works.
- Discuss team goals and expectations.

Ask, "Why are you here?" I used this question to emphasize the answer: there is a place for everyone, even non-runners coming in, as long as they are willing to work. I gave the example of a freshman who had never run, was involved with martial arts, and her neighbor said to join up for fun, meet good people, and get out of regular physical education class. This runner became the number one runner at UCLA several years later! (See the Case Study on Bronte Golick earlier.)

For the next part of the meeting, I sent the newcomers outside with the captains for a "getting to know you" session. Meanwhile, the parents remained in the room to hear from the parent and Booster Club leaders about how they could become involved in and support the team. They would hear about financial issues and opportunities to help at meets, pre-meet dinners, and the end of the season awards banquet.

Let me take a moment to discuss the role of assistant coaches. I am aware that in many smaller programs, there may not be an assistant coach. Some programs may not have a paid assistant coach but instead, have volunteers fill the role of supporting the head coach. I believe there are some key things to consider when hiring and working with an assistant. Let me cover those here.

It is important for the assistant to be a runner. Then, they understand running and can run with the athletes, which is helpful for safety and supervision. Can a non-runner be an assistant coach? If they were formally a runner and currently have injuries that prevent running but encourage the person to ride a bike alongside the runners—that is an adequate second choice.

As I have explained, I mainly coached female runners and found it very helpful to have a female assistant coach. The athletes were comforted by the presence of a coach who could understand the issues unique to their gender. It makes the parents of female athletes more confident when there is a same-gender coach involved in the program.

Having knowledge of the sport, beyond just as a participant, is certainly preferable. I would suggest that if you, as the head coach are experienced and knowledgeable, then the assistant does not necessarily need to be an expert. If, on the other hand, you are new to this, having an assistant with expertise can be very important.

Make sure that you are very clear with the assistant during the interview and hiring process about what is expected of them. Go over the hours and days they are expected to come to practices and attend meets. Provide them with a calendar and schedule. Be clear about any paperwork to be filled out. They may be required to pass certain certification tests as required by the school. Often needed is a current certification in first aid and cardiopulmonary resuscitation (CPR). The school or district may require fingerprinting and tuberculosis testing. It is your responsibility as head coach to ensure all of these requirements are fulfilled by your new assistant.

Discuss your philosophy of coaching and training with the assistant. It should be clear what duties and responsibilities you see them fulfilling as the assistant. Talk about how, and when, you want input from them regarding the program. Will they be a partner with equal input into decisions? Or will they follow your lead and support your choices as head coach?

Here is a list of jobs you may want to have your assistant do for you and the team:
- Supervision of drills, practice runs, and team meetings
- Data collection during workouts and races
- Assistance with injury assessment and rehabilitation of injured athletes
- Liaison with captains and other team leaders

- Consult with you, the head coach, regarding race lineups and workouts per your procedure
- Be responsible for a particular group or portion of the team (for example the freshman or junior varsity)

CHAPTER 10:

BOOSTER CLUB AND PARENT INVOLVEMENT

Your Program Support System

I used to say, "The athletes and coaches are the team, but the parents and families make it a program," Parent involvement in a positive way, of course, is crucial to the success of the program. There are so many things that a positive, active group of parents can do to make the life of the coach easier. They can make it possible for the coach to focus on the technical aspects of running workouts, also known as the "x"s and "o"s. Over the years at Capistrano Valley High School, we developed an extraordinarily strong, active, and supportive Booster Club. Several coaches from outside our program were amazed at how organized and productive the parent organization was. They could not believe all that the parents did, and, therefore, what I did not have to do, allowing me to properly coach the athletes.

I have heard some coaches lament the involvement of parents in their program. They are reluctant to have a Booster Club for fear of losing control or of possible parent interference. I never found this to be a problem. The overwhelming amount of work provided by the Booster Club far outweighed any minor negative consequences. Perhaps I was lucky in having such great parents over the years who so selflessly contributed to the work of this program. I literally could not have accomplished what I did with my teams without those dedicated parents.

Our Booster Club was organized and run to benefit *both* the boys' and girls' teams.

Once again, you need to be aware of what rules and requirements there may be for establishing a Booster Club at your school and in your district, region, and state. At CVHS, it was necessary to establish a formal organization under federal Internal Revenue Service guidelines. There had to be by-laws written and approved by the school and school district. Elections had to be held to establish the officers. One of the main concerns was how money was handled and accounted for. We have all, unfortunately, heard of too many occasions where money for Little League or non-school soccer programs was mishandled. In fact, even with the by-laws and rules in place, an elected treasurer, who was a parent of a boys' team member, embezzled money. Fortunately, after a year of working with law enforcement, much of the money was recovered. However, it caused us to reevaluate some of our procedures, including requiring dual signatures on checks, which I recommend for added security.

There are certainly many ways that parents can be involved and different ways to organize them. Our Booster Club developed over many years in an organic way. As has been a common theme throughout this book, I will explain my own experience to provide you with a starting point. You may have different needs and requirements that may cause your Booster Club to be organized differently. You need to find the unique way that best serves the needs of your team.

Certainly, fundraising is a key aspect of any school athletic team these days. Schools, districts, and states may have quite different ways to fund athletic teams. Briefly, CVHS—in conjunction with the Capistrano Unified School District (CUSD)—only paid for one head coach per gender and no assistants. If an on-campus classroom teacher was the coach, he or she received a class period that corresponded with the assigned athletics time slot. So in my case, I taught four academic classes and had a cross-country class (track in the spring) as my fifth class period of assigned work.

CVHS and CUSD paid for some of our entry fees for meets but not all. They provided buses to meets upon request. Little if any money was provided for equipment. Assistant coaches had to be paid for with money raised by the Booster Club.

It is important to note that in California, under rules established in a legal decision, schools cannot require athletes to pay for anything. A team can request or encourage donations, but schools cannot require payment in exchange for participation. Therefore, fundraising is particularly difficult.

At our Newcomers Meeting, the Booster Club leaders would attempt to educate the new parents about the realities of team financing without scaring them off. In general, a requested donation of approximately $125–$150 per athlete was established for the summer training portion of the season. This was primarily to pay for coaches. For the actual season, mid-August into November, we asked for $250 per athlete. Families with multiple participants were offered discounts. The fall season donations helped pay for assistant coaches, the banquet, awards, pre-meet dinners, food at meets, and some equipment. T-shirts and uniforms were provided by the Boosters, although uniforms could be purchased if athletes did not want to have to borrow and return a loaner. Several fundraisers were also tried over the years, some more successful than others. Among them were dine-out opportunities where the team received a portion of the proceeds, collection of shoes for disadvantaged youth, which we were provided some funds for gathering, raffles, and sale of "gold cards" or coupon packages. More recently, the Boosters began a golf tournament that raised a significant amount of money through the greens' fees for participating golfers, a silent auction at the post-golf dinner, and a ball drop where athletes sold chances at having the closest ball to the hole after a helicopter dropped balls onto the green!

The Booster Club held a meeting early in the summer for parents and athletes. Athletes were able to try on and order uniforms and t-shirts. Athletes also had the option to buy other gear (sweats, gym bags, backpacks, and pajamas) that made the team made some money. At this meeting, parents were presented with a variety of options for participation in support of the team.

Among these were:

- Hosting pre-meet dinners
- Providing a portion of the meal at pre-meet dinners
- Providing fruit, bagels, and drinks at meets
- Working on the end-of-year banquet—this had many jobs associated with it
- Creating photo albums for each athlete with pictures featuring them for the season necessitated at least eight photographers organized by gender and grade
- Transporting the tents, tarps, coolers, and tables to meets
- Helping order and distribute t-shirts, uniforms, sweats, and other swag

CHAPTER 11:

SCHOOL ADMINISTRATION

The support of the school administration is important. This needs to be cultivated so that your program receives the maximum support possible—be it financial or practical.

The athletic director (AD) is a key person to support a strong program. They are involved in hiring assistants, equipment purchases, possible financial support for meets, and clearing (explanation below) your athletes for participation. The AD may schedule the buses, handle coaching payroll, and aid with awards at the end of the season. They may also be of great help in publicizing your sport from weekly shout-outs about team and individual accomplishments, to recruitment at feeder schools, as discussed earlier. Additionally, the AD may be the person responsible for your use of facilities on campus. A good relationship with your AD is also helpful when and if there are concerns about your program brought to the administration by parents or athletes.

Here are some more details on how the AD can support you and your program:

- Scheduling your athletic team in the school master schedule for the appropriate class period or after school.
- Hiring assistants, checking credentials and references, and arranging for district approval of hires.
- Informing you and your assistants with updates and guidance of various certifications that you may be required to have—*e.g.*, first aid, concussion protocols, and heat-related issues. Many of these are done through National Federation of State High School Associations (NFHS). Visit their website for courses and certificates available.
- Arranging for, approving of, and perhaps paying for, purchases. You need to make sure that you follow the correct procedures in purchasing equipment. Do not assume you will get reimbursed. Check with the AD. Do not use funds given to you for donations to buy equipment unless authorized.
- Paying entry fees for meets and invitationals. At CVHS, the procedure was that I provided the AD a copy of the meet fees at least two weeks prior to when I needed the check.
- Arranging for transportation. The AD was the one I went through to request buses for transport to meets. This was often done months ahead of time. Make sure you know who to go to and especially the timeline required to make those requests.
- The AD or another administrator, may be the person who handles requests and scheduling of on campus facilities, like the track, pool, and the weight room.
- Find out who can post information about schedules, results, and other information on the school website. At CVHS, the Athletic Department had a school-wide website where each sport could post information, results, schedules, and (with proper consent) pictures.

- An especially important function of the AD was the handling of the clearance process for individual athletes to participate. This may vary among districts and states, but it usually involves the athlete and parents providing proof of a recent physical exam, a copy of an insurance card, and many signature pages regarding conduct and liability. Usually, athletes are not allowed to participate in meets, maybe not even practices, until these forms are turned in and approved by the AD or other appropriate official.

In addition to the AD, many schools have a separate position: activities director. This administrator at CVHS dealt more with non-sports activities, like pep rallies and dances, but still had a role on the financial side of sports, such as requests for spending funds. In addition, this may be the site of the office or person who provides school-wide publicity about your sport.

Most schools have some form of daily announcements over loudspeakers, printed, posted online, or televised. Make sure that you do as much as possible to get your team and individuals in the school news. Athletes love to be recognized by their peers who might not be on the team. It is also a good way to bring positive publicity to your program and therefore recruit athletes.

It is important to cultivate a good relationship with the Guidance Office. At CVHS, the assistant principal (in charge of the scheduling), the registrar, and individual guidance counselors had the latest roster and athlete schedule information. When conflicts arose between academic classes and the athletic periods, the people in the Guidance Office are the ones who helped resolve those conflicts.

CHAPTER 12:

CAPTAIN-AND ATHLETE-LED PRACTICES

Leadership in Action

I n California, there are rules preventing coaches in all sports from directly coaching the skills of the sport for a period of two to three weeks, usually at some point prior to the start of the training and competing cycle. This is referred to as the "dead period." Most cross-country coaches choose to take this period right at the end of school/track season so they can use the summer to build up consecutive weeks of workouts without interruption. To determine the beginning of coach-led formal summer practices, I counted twenty or twenty-one weeks backward from the State Meet (the Saturday after Thanksgiving) to establish the start of coach-led practices. At CVHS, as in most programs, a period of athlete-led practices usually preceded the formal coach-led practices. This helped me comply with the rules, as well as provide adequate rest for the runners following the end of the track season. Additionally, I used the dead period personally for travel and vacation, given that during most of my coaching career, my wife and I were both teachers. This provided an opportunity for us to get away without interfering with the upcoming summer training season and coaching.

Our school year class schedule ran from late August to early June. Our season began with meets in early September with our State Meet, as mentioned above, happening just after Thanksgiving. As a coach, you need to determine several things as you set up your dead period. You need to determine how many weeks your overall macro cycle of training is, from the last meet back to your first practice. The answer, of course, is rooted in your philosophy of training. I like a total of twenty-four weeks. This put our first captain-led practice somewhere in middle to late June.

Under a strict interpretation of the CIF rules regarding the dead period, I did not participate in planning, directing, or implementing those athlete-, or captain-led, practices. They were run strictly by the captains. All athletes, veterans, and newcomers alike were provided with guidelines in the late spring for how to build up their mileage to be prepared to begin coach-led practices in July.

Captains demonstrated the right warmup, cool-down, and stretch-down routines. They were aware about making sure that newcomers were well cared for and welcomed by veteran runners. Top veterans sometimes sacrificed their own run on a particular day to stay with slower girls going shorter distances than the vets may have been capable of. The purpose of this was to have the veterans nurture and encourage the newcomers. These veterans sometimes then did a second workout later or followed with more running after the formal practice was concluded to achieve their own pace or mileage goals. These captain/athlete-led practices were a great chance for athletes to develop chemistry and bond without the coach. Picking good captains, therefore, is a key to this phase of training.

Captains: Selection and Duties

There are a wide variety of methods for picking captains and an even wider variety of ways coaches make use of captains. I am going to share with you my approach and rationale.

I never had athlete-selected captains. I felt like this lent itself too much to a popularity contest, and the result could have been captains that perhaps were mismatched with each other or with the coach. I believed that captains rose to the forefront over their years in the program. It became obvious who they were, for they were the leaders. I never had a set number of captains. I usually only had seniors as captains—and those who almost always had started with my program as freshmen or at least by the time they were sophomores. By the time, these runners were seniors with three or four years of experience on my teams, they stood out as leaders. They developed naturally, and their interaction with their teammates showcased their leadership qualities. I selected anywhere from two to six captains with an average of four.

The captains were not just the fastest runners, though certainly, one or two of them were likely to be. Sometimes, the fastest might be an underclass person (lucky for you!). I tried to ensure that a non-varsity captain would represent the non-varsity runners and share their concerns.

The assistant coaches and I met with the captains after they were selected to go over their roles and responsibilities. We encouraged them to bring new ideas and approaches to the table for discussion and possible implementation.

Basic captain duties included:
- Start practice by leading warmup runs and daily drills.

- Help to organize workout groups during the key part of the workout.
- Act as a liaison between coaches and athletes.
- Represent the team at pep rallies and assemblies.
- Organize social and bonding activities, such as "secret sisters" (explained later).
- Present special awards to team members for their effort or times after meets.

CHAPTER 13:

SETTING UP THE SUMMER PROGRAM

Organizing for Winning

I n this chapter, I will discuss the overall approach to the summer but not the specific workouts since those were covered in the earlier chapters. I remind you here of the previous discussion to be aware of any rules regarding training and coach-athlete contact in the summertime.

At your Newcomers Meeting and in communications with your returning veterans, you need to establish clear guidelines regarding the athletes' responsibilities in preparation for the summer. Explain how much you want them to run: how often, how far, and how fast. Will you have rules or requirements for how much they have done or can do by the first coach-led practice? For example, my runners, needed to be able to run four miles without stopping by the first coach-led practice in mid-July. As mentioned previously, this would have followed a three-week captain-led period, during which they were doing three or four workouts a week.

I created a handout that I posted on the team website titled, "Preparing for Summer Practices." It was a bit tongue-in-cheek, initially, with a section called "How to Get Injured, Sick, Perform Poorly, and Get So Discouraged You Want to Quit." I went on to say get up as late as possible so you do not have blood flow to muscles and do not have time to properly hydrate and eat. Then in all seriousness, I suggested that athletes wake up at least an hour and a half before practice time, along with how much to eat and drink, and how much fluid to bring to practice (see the discussion of nutrition and hydration for details).

Depending on the rules of your school, you may or may not be able to make summer participation a mandatory part of the athletic grade for cross country. I could not do so because the class of "cross country" did not officially begin until school was in session. If you are able to base grades on summer participation, you must establish and clearly communicate how that is going to be done. Is it by the number of workouts attended? Is it how many miles run? Is there some time standard to be met? To be on the team, I made the requirement to complete a five-mile run in fifty minutes or six miles in sixty-five minutes. Let me point out that anyone not able to do so had almost always dropped out over the summer anyway. Those were not tough standards in my region or for our levels of competitive preparation. (See the **Resources** page for suggested pre-summer miles build-up.)

I also required a specific minimum number of documented miles run during the summer to be considered for competing in the first race of the season. This served two defensible purposes. The first was a safety preparedness argument. Athletes would more likely have an injury-free, safe, and healthy first race if they met this minimum requirement. Second, requiring a minimum amount of running mileage meant regular participation. For example, if my summer program, including the captain-led period, lasted twelve weeks and ended with the first race of the season, then a minimum requirement of 250–275 miles was my standard. My teams certainly had top girls running twice that mileage and more. (See **Resources** for a sample of daily/ weekly miles spreadsheet.)

This leads to a discussion about tryouts or time trials to make the team. There are many approaches regarding this topic, and all have as many good points as bad ones. I did not require a time trial to be on the team. Early in my career, there were too many examples of athletes who would not have been on the team at all had there been a time trial. They became varsity-level runners—or at least very solid members of the team—who loved running and contributed much to the program. I was told by several of my coaching colleagues that I could not be really successful unless I implemented a time trial. Their reasoning was that it caused the athletes to be more serious about the summer training and eliminated those who might not take running seriously, would become a drag on the program, and take up valuable coaching time with excuses and injuries. These coaches would require something like a 24:30 time for three miles for freshman or newcomer girls and 21:30 or faster for freshman or newcomer boys. Again, I think this shortchanges future solid runners and eliminates them too quickly. In addition, my colleagues were concerned about the need to reduce the gap between the faster and slower runners because they thought it was too hard to coach such a wide range of abilities. I did not find this to be a valid concern, at least for me and my system.

As you will recall from the details of the training system, each athlete had an individualized training goal for each workout based on previous workout data. Calculation of the goal per runner does take some time to do, but to be honest, it is one of the reasons I had so much success at *all* levels. I provided personalized workouts for each and every runner, regardless of ability. They all felt special, and they all could improve at appropriate personal rates. I do remember some snarky joy in holding the second of two consecutive—and much coveted—Orange County Championship trophies, while pointing out to one of those coaching colleagues that, indeed, I still did not have any time trials or tryouts!

You need to determine how formally your summer program will be structured. This may be determined by your school, district, or state rules. Make sure you understand what permits, facilities requests, and insurance issues may be involved. In my case, I used a variety of sites away from the school campus during the summer since we would be stuck at school during the academic year. At one park, I just needed a simple form and a common understanding with the ranger. At another, I needed to file quite a bit of paperwork and get proof of insurance coverage by the school district . . . and that was just for three dates in the summertime.

Are you going to be charging a fee for the summer training? This may be a function of your school and district rules and procedures. In some areas, coaches may run camps on their own, charge fees as they wish, and pay facilities and insurance costs generated from their income. In California public schools, we could not charge fees but rather request donations. Our district eventually went to a system where coaches had to run all finances through the school site activities office. We could charge student-athletes what was needed to raise the money to pay coaches' salaries and various other fees. Coach pay was tied to the pay scale negotiated between the district and the teachers' union. Our summer donation varied from $125–$175, depending on the year. That paid for coaches' salaries and some minor equipment. Coaches were not paid by the school or district for the summer training and was the responsibility of the Booster Clubs.

Many programs, ours included, provided a big end-of-summer event. This could be a workout followed by food and a program meeting with parents and athletes of both boys' and girls' teams. It creates an opportunity to celebrate the end of summer and prepare everyone for the beginning of the competitive season. In my program, we called it "The Beach Run."

The Beach Run was an incredibly fun tradition. It began with a Saturday long run. The course wound through Laguna Niguel and Dana Point, finishing at Doheny Beach Park. There, parents, and families would await the athletes as they arrived and cheered them into a grassy finish area. Athletes were assigned different lengths of runs corresponding to their fitness levels, with the goal of trying to have all athletes arrive at relatively the same time. Parents supervised the entire route, gave directions, provided drinks, and followed on bikes, in cars, or ran themselves to ensure the safety for all of the runners. Following a regular stretch-down routine, athletes and parents then enjoyed a meal prepared by the Booster Club. For many years, it was a complete barbeque, but that transformed to a simpler post-run meal: bagel, toast, fruit, and lots of sports drinks and water.

After the food, a meeting for parents was held where coaches and Boosters Club members spoke on a variety of topics pertinent to the beginning of the racing season, which usually began the following week. At that time, uniforms, t-shirts, sweats, and sweat bags were passed out to those who pre-ordered them. The biggest Beach Run in my career was attended by eighty girls and seventy guy runners and families. There were over 400 participants! The Beach Run was a highlight of the summer season. If you can think of some way to do something similar at your school, I think you will find great benefits in team-building and enthusiasm for parents, families, and athletes.

To sum up the summer program: decide what kind of program you will have, investigate what rules apply, and learn how the financing works. Determine and communicate to athletes what goals and expectations you have for them.

Rise and shine; it is running time! Get running!

CASE STUDY: CARLY CORSINITA
From Humble Beginnings to the Oregon Ducks . . . Because She Wanted It

Carly Corsinita, now of the University of Oregon Ducks cross country and track and field teams certainly did not start out headed that way. Carly arrived for her freshman summer workouts in July of 2017 with little running background, a tiny body, and a wide-eyed look way up to the tall, lean senior, Haley Herberg, who would be California State Champion and NXN finalist in a few months. Her freshman season developed steadily, if not unremarkably with her finishing that year with a best time of 19:30.

However, during the track and field season that followed, wherever Herberg and Alyssa Bautista, a Footlocker finalist went, Carly followed. When they were blazing a distance run at 7:10 pace, she was keeping up as long as she could. When they were rocking 400s on the track at ridiculous paces, Carly was trying to match them. Not wanting to rain on her parade, I cautiously asked if she was doing okay and whether or not she might be overdoing it, trying to keep up with these national-caliber girls. She explained that she wanted to be as good as they were and accomplish what they had accomplished. She knew the way to do that was to do what they were doing. So she did!

By the end of her sophomore cross-country season, she had dropped her personal record (PR) to 17:31. Her junior season saw her become one of the leading girls in Southern California with a PR of 16:54. During her junior season at track and field, she just missed the State Meet, which she did make as a senior. By the time her senior year of cross country was finished, Carly was a multiple-league and county champion and the Orange County Register Cross Country "Runner of the Year," something her mentor and model, Haley Herberg, had also achieved.

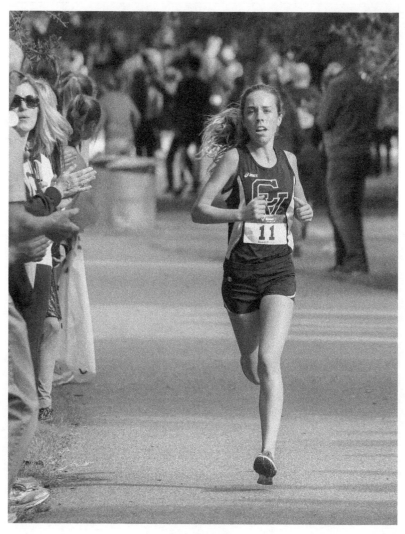

Carly Corsinita

Carly finished her career with personal bests of 4:58 at 1600, 10:29 at 3200, and 16:54 at the three miles cross-country distance. Her three sub-seventeen-minute races and ten sub-17:20 performances earned her a trip to Eugene as an Oregon Duck. All this was accomplished because she wanted it to happen and was willing to do the hard work to make it a reality.

CASE STUDY: JVS AND OTHER NON-VARSITY RUNNERS
Unsung Heroes, Future Stars, and Lifelong Runners

As the 2014 season began, Kelsie King was a senior on the Capistrano Valley High School cross-country team and expected to be in the top ten of what experts projected to be (and eventually was) a top team in the state and nation.

As the season began to unfold and Kelsie's work ethic and dedication improved her times, she was in a position to run in a couple of varsity races when those ahead of her were injured, ill, or just needed to some rest. When a formerly-injured girl, returned and ran well at League Finals, Kelsie became an alternate as the top ten girls (only seven to race) moved on to post-season competition. When one of the varsity girls struggled at CIFSS Prelims, Kelsie took her place at CIFSS Finals and helped the team to a second-place finish and another trip to the State Championships where she competed very well. This earned her a scholarship to a Division 2 school in the Midwest.

Kelsie was prepared, and it paid off.

If you coach a runner—or are that runner—who is not yet one of the top athletes, or like Kelsie, on the edge of the varsity team, revisit the case studies included in this book on Carly Corsinita and Bronte Golick. Neither started out on top. Through hard work and dedication, they each became stars and future college runners, but they did not start out that way.

Remember that it takes a lot of runners to make a team successful. Most coaches do not measure their overall programs' success just on the accomplishments of the varsity team. Junior varsity (JV) teams in California are made up of juniors and seniors who are not on varsity and then there are age group teams for sophomores and freshman. In some states or regions, there may be just varsity, and then everyone else is on JV. Each of these teams needs five runners to score in meets and so on most teams, especially smaller ones, everyone may be important to the team's success.

At Capistrano Valley High, we took pride in how well our non-varsity teams did. Between 2012 and 2018, at our peak, our non-varsity teams won more plaques and trophies for team performances than any other program in our area of Orange County, one of the most competitive in the nation.

Train up! That is, challenge yourself to run with someone faster than you, like Carly Corsinita did in the case study mentioned earlier. If you are studying or using the VDOT training system I described previously, then find the workout paces just above your current level. As you continually train up, you will speed up; it is just that simple.

Being a distance runner has many benefits. You learn and practice discipline, hard work, dedication, and teamwork. You build confidence and learn what it means to contribute to something greater than you. I have had more non-varsity runners become lifelong runners than varsity athletes.

I believe this is because they learned to genuinely appreciate the joy of running and the rewards of challenging themselves to be better.

CHAPTER 14:

SELECT SUMMER TRAINING CAMPS

Mammoth Camp

Many teams hold special summer training camps away from the campus. These camps can serve many purposes from team bonding to extra educational and training opportunities. Often, these camps are held at high-altitude vacation or resort areas to provide challenging workouts as well as recreational activities and team fun. A note regarding high-altitude training: the physiological benefits of training at altitude cannot be achieved in a week. It takes three weeks or more for the improvement in performance as a result of high-altitude training to take place. High-altitude training for a week should be viewed as a challenge to be met and shared, not a scientifically-based method to improve cardiovascular fitness. Some coaches offer programs to all athletes who are interested, others have tryouts or selection processes and take only the best and the fittest of the runners.

In California, many teams go to Mammoth Mountain/Mammoth Lakes in the Eastern High Sierra for special summer training camps. In July and early August there may be twenty or more high school and college teams staying and training in the area. This is also where the Mammoth Track Club trains—with many professionals on the streets, in the parks, and on the trails. The altitude of the city where many of the condos are located is at roughly 7,500 feet with surrounding trails, peaks, and lakes well over 10,000 feet. Some teams camp, but most stay in some of the many condos offered at a wide range of rates. There are some good deals in what, for Mammoth, is the off-season (from the ski season).

I took teams to Mammoth for over twenty years. Originally, I took all runners, but too many newcomers turned out to be unprepared, and some veterans wanted to go only for the fun and less for the training. I eventually used an invitation-only model. I developed a comprehensive spreadsheet (see **Resources**) that constantly updated and compared data until selection time came. I would factor the previous years' team ranking, the track distance ranking, captain-led practice attendance, miles run, and attendance over the first several weeks of coach-led summer practice, as well as paces, for as many measured runs as I could get in prior to selection time. Generally, I would invite between sixteen and twenty-two athletes, depending on the number of volunteer adult drivers and rooms. Team captains attended automatically if they were healthy.

The coaches and volunteer parents who drove stayed in one larger condo that was also used as home base for the team meetings and dining area. Athletes usually stayed in three other rooms of various sizes. A captain or two were in each room and helped me put together the room assignments. Since we usually went in early to mid-August, we had to get rooms booked by April. Some years, we rented a large van, supplemented by other coach or parent vehicles. In the last few years, there were many parent volunteers who did the driving. This saved the team money.

For camp purposes, make sure you educate yourself about any paperwork your school or district may require. For CVHS, I had to fill out a comprehensive Field Study request, get permission slips and medical and liability clearances, and submit the request several months ahead of time (before the start of summer) for approval. Adult drivers had to fill out forms and provide proof of insurance, as well. In the package for athletes and parents was a guide to room rules and behavior expectations that both parents and athletes were required to agree to and sign.

Under California rules, I was not allowed to charge a fee, and no one could be denied access to camp due to lack of funds. To counter this, I requested a $300 donation from each runner in the last several years. Fortunately, I had a 90–95 percent donation rate. This covered condo rentals, food and beverages, gasoline for all drivers, and a small administrative fee for the coach. Some coaches charge more and make more, and others charge less. Ultimately, that is up to you, your school, and your parents. Medical insurance considerations can vary from place to place, so make sure you are clear about whether you will need to provide it. In my case, since it was a school function, the school and district covered the insurance. Most coaches also carry some insurance policies through various coaching associations such as the National Federation of High School Associations (NFHS).

Some teams go to camp for a full week, some a bit less. My camp was four nights and five days. Our participants met in the school parking lot and left at 7:00 a.m. on Wednesday morning, arriving at a park near the entrance to town by 2:00 p.m. An introductory workout took place from that spot before going to the rooms to unload and then get ready for dinner.

The first workout at altitude is a challenge, and it is important to make sure the athletes know this ahead of time so as not to be discouraged and/or overdo the workout. Also, take some time to educate about altitude sickness and the impact of altitude on paces and abilities. Hydration is particularly important at altitude, so be sure athletes are hydrating on the drive up before that first workout begins.

The typical workout schedule for our camp would look like this:

- Wednesday afternoon: 35–45-minute run.
- Thursday morning: 50–60-minute run.
- Thursday afternoon: 25–30-minute run.
- Friday morning: Hike. Often, we drove an hour up into the Tuolumne Meadows High Country of Yosemite National Park. We did a four-to-five-hour aggressive hike at high altitude (10,000–11,000 feet), which gets the heart rate up like a flat land run! We then stopped at a lake for lunch with options to swim and sunbathe before returning.
- Friday afternoon: 25–30-minute run.
- Saturday morning: 65–75-minute long run.
- Saturday afternoon: 30-minute pool work with yoga and stretching recovery.
- Sunday morning: no workout, just preparing to leave. According to CIF rules, we were not allowed to conduct organized workouts on Sunday.

It is important to communicate to the athletes the impact of altitude. I found that even state-champion-level runners were slower at altitude. I calculated that twenty to forty-five seconds a mile slower was a good general guideline to compare times to flat land running paces. If an athlete who normally ran an eight-minute pace for six miles on flat land at no altitude ran for forty-eight minutes at 8000 feet of elevation, they may only cover five or five and a half miles. So, I converted their miles run at altitude to a flat land equivalent for each runner to make it clear what they were accomplishing compared to those at home.

It is important, prior to leaving for camp, to establish clear rules about behavior and expectations on any road trip or overnight function. I had all athletes and parents agree to a set of room rules, which were consistent with the school discipline plan. Here is what that looked like:

- This is a *team and school* trip, not a vacation.
- *Everything* you say and do is a reflection on your school, coaches, and parents.
- This is a school activity, so all school rules apply. There is zero tolerance for alcohol and drugs.
- There is no "I" in TEAM so place the interests of the team above your own. Be a positive force; work with all.
- Remember, we have a diverse group; be respectful of those who are different than you.
- Be considerate to all teammates, coaches, and parents.
- Be in your rooms by curfew and stay there unless specifically allowed by coaches or parents.
- If it is a co-ed trip, you may not be in rooms with the opposite sex.
- Designated lights-out time needs to be strictly observed. As athletes you need rest, and you need to respect the fact that your teammates need sleep and rest, too.
- Be on time to all scheduled activities.
- Respect and take care of hotels, condos, and camps.
- Do not gossip. It is hurtful and does not promote a positive team atmosphere.

- Whenever you see, hear, or experience something going on that you feel is not right, contact a coach or parent immediately.
- NO INITIATION OR HAZING RITUALS ARE ALLOWED. If you would not be comfortable describing it to your grandma or the school principal, DON'T DO IT.

Athletes were assigned to kitchen duty in a rotating fashion that intentionally paired them with different teammates from different rooms each time to promote team bonding and chemistry. Meal prep and cleanup were done by the athletes with coach and adult supervision. I experimented over the years with different menus. Prior to camp, I would ask athletes if hey had any particular dietary restrictions. I eventually settled one that was easy to prepare, inexpensive, and healthy.

Breakfast consisted of healthy cereals, yogurt, fruit, toast, bagels, and energy bars. Lunch was making your own sandwiches with lunch meat, peanut butter and jelly, chips, fruits, veggies, and nuts. Dinners included build your own burrito/taco bowls and salads, pasta nights, burgers (veggie included), and make your own pizza night. Snacks and desserts were available. What eventually developed among the athletes was a custom of bringing some of their own snacks and supplements to meals. You may choose to discourage, forbid, allow, or encourage snacks as you see fit with your program.

As part of the camp experience, I included several educational seminars—usually two per day. Sometimes, they were led by assistant coaches or the athletes themselves. Topics included: diet and nutrition, explanation of the science of training, developing racing goals for the season, racing tactics, scoring strategies, and review of upcoming race courses and opponents. These were usually done following some getting to know you, team-bonding activity that took ten to twenty minutes. The seminars lasted forty-five minutes to an hour. This was also a time when outside videos, books, and articles were presented.

Of course, a variety of talent shows, skits, and team-building activities can and should be incorporated in the camp schedule to make it fun and encourage that all-important team chemistry.

CHAPTER 15:

THE PROMISED LAND

Post-Season Championship Racing

I remember the first time we made the California State Championships as a team in 2012.

The sheer joy our runners and families experienced that morning at Mount San Antonio College is one of my greatest memories as a coach. We had done it! The planning, goal setting, and hard work had paid off with our trip to the promised land: Woodward Park in Fresno, California.

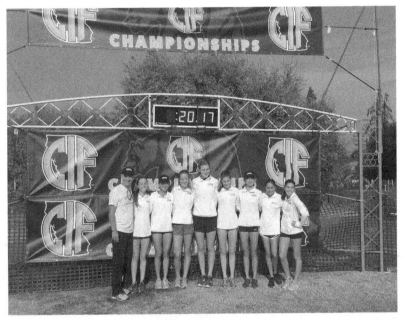

State meet team, 2017

The California State Championship is considered the most difficult high school state race to qualify for and the most competitive in the nation. And we were going. It would be the first of six straight team trips and two additional trips with a top individual. In 2014, we were one of two teams nationwide considered for the final at-large spot for NXN in Portland. Unfortunately, we were not chosen, but it was certainly nice to be considered. This helped establish the CVHS program as a California State powerhouse.

There are some unique things to consider once you get to the post-season. In this chapter, I offer some ideas. First, let me point out what happens in California since I will be referring to those meets in my examples and schedule. Then, I will discuss the continued training, followed by the sensitive issues of team selection, and finally some practical considerations regarding travel.

California is divided into ten sections, each governed by state guidelines. The rules allow some room to organize the section championships in the way that best fits the sections' needs and numbers. CVHS is in the Southern Section, which is the largest and includes almost half of all the schools in the state—well over 500 schools.

Our post-season began after qualifying from our league, the South Coast League. Next came the first round of the playoffs, CIF-Southern Section (SS) Prelims. The state and its ten sections are divided into five divisions, which are based on student enrollment. In our CIF-SS Prelims, our team was likely to be in a heat (one of three or four) with sixteen to twenty teams attempting to qualify to be in the final sixteen to twenty teams—depending on the year and specific number of schools competing. When the CIF-SS Finals were held, the state rules determined that seven teams from each of the five divisions in the Southern Section would qualify for the State Meet. There is a formula for individual qualifiers (without their teams) at each of the levels, from League to Prelims and Finals to the State Meet.

Certainly, the twenty plus boys' and twenty plus girls' teams in each of the five divisions and the individuals who earn spots to compete in the California State Cross Country Championships are among the nation's best. Many of the teams and individuals are nationally ranked. The competition is at a premium on the 5k course at Woodward Park. Many future Olympians and elite professional runners compete and win there. I was fortunate enough to coach an individual State Champion, Haley Herberg, currently at the University of Washington (2020), where, as referenced earlier, she won the Pac-12 individual title in March 2021. She covered the moderate 5k course in seventeen minutes flat, one of the top ten times in California State Meet history.

In reviewing the training cycle at this point, remember that the schedule is unique to California. Our meets start much later in the year than other parts of the country due to weather considerations. First meets in California are not held until early September and the Southern Section Prelims and Finals are held on consecutive weeks in mid-November. The State Meet immediately follows on the Saturday of Thanksgiving weekend. Check the calendar for your state if you are not from California.

Let me remind you of my "Training" chapter, where I explain that in order to start training, you must determine when you will finish your season and then plan backward. For CVHS, counting back from the State Meet, the athlete-/captain-led training began in mid- to late June, and coach-led practices (under CIF rules) began in mid-July. I previously indicated a three-week peaking and tapering period is appropriate prior to the California State Meet, and ours actually began *after* our League Championship Meet. As you can see from the previously detailed weekly and daily workout schedules, my runners were working hard, even while trying to qualify in our League, to get into the playoffs. This feat was a big challenge since our league, the South Coast League, was considered among the toughest, if not *the* toughest in California. Runners must have a lot of confidence and preparation to be able to get out of the South Coast League and to CIF Prelims.

I remember posting a question/comment on PrepCalTrack's website about a "nice problem to have"—specifically, how to decide which of my many deserving runners would comprise the team moving on to the CIF competition. Of course, only seven runners can race, and there were no other races for the rest of the team to compete in at this time. Standard procedure in our area was to have between ten and twelve runners make up your CIF team. While the rest of the team began the off-season, these CIF runners continued to train for the next three weeks in preparation for the State Meet. Sometimes, the top seven racers would be obvious, but more commonly, it was uncertain. This was an extremely difficult decision to make.

Some coaches just go by their instinct. Some favor experience and seniority; others actually take talented youth over seniority on the grounds that they will run the following season. Should consideration be given to who is hot? What about the course demands? Is one athlete better suited to the specific race course? All of these were factors in the selection.

Unfortunately, these choices are a source of *lots* of tension and anxiety for the athletes, parents, and coaches. Athletes want to be a part of these races. It may help them earn college entrance. Parents want their kids to do these races and can be narrow-sighted in their view of who deserves to be racing. I am not good with conflict, and these kinds of pressures can be particularly draining. To be honest, some of the great joy of accomplishment during these peak State Championship years was somewhat diminished by the anguish of deciding the lineup each week. There were hurt feelings no matter how thoughtfully and thoroughly I considered this issue.

Develop protocols for making the decision process clear and transparent. Some coaches have developed a ranking system with points. This could include seniority, most recent race results, an injury factor, and a consideration for the course(s). However you decide to do this, make the protocols clear and put them in writing prior to the beginning of the season. Reiterate, prior to the championship phase, how the process will be followed so there are no misunderstandings. Express to parents and athletes your understanding of how difficult this is for everybody. Perhaps consider having parents and athletes sign something prior to the start of the season that acknowledges their understanding of how the choices will be determined, including an agreement that they will accept the choices.

Travel to away meets, especially championship ones, should be a cause for joy and celebration. In most cases, the key here is planning ahead. My Booster parents would book rooms for the State Meet in

May, six months prior to the November races. We would leave on the Friday morning after Thanksgiving and drive five hours to Woodward Park in Fresno, California. After some swag shopping and photo opportunities at the finish line, it was time for our pre-meet routine out on the course itself. Fortunately, many of our runners had been on the course before, either at previous State Meets and or at an invitational held there in October, where many top teams go with the intention of practicing on the State Meet course. We would check in at the hotel, shower, and head out for a meal together with families, athletes, and coaches. Reservations are certainly necessary months ahead of time for hotels and restaurants.

The CVHS Booster Club paid for the rooms and dinner for coaches and athletes. Parents and family members paid their own way.

State Meet race day is a truly glorious experience, and, of course, I am biased about the California State Meet being the best of the best. It is important that you and your athletes make sure to enjoy each moment—from the time you do your pre-meet routines to, hopefully, being on the podium as a winning team at the end of your race. The first time at a State Meet can be intimidating, even overwhelming. It is your job as the coach to help runners and parents alike to stay in the moment.

Keep your routines, pre-meet and warmup drills, all the same. Do not try anything new. Then *enjoy*!

CHAPTER 16:

AWARDS AND REWARDS

Recognition of a Job Well Done

I t is essential to keep the runners in a positive mindset. One of the best ways to achieve this is through a variety of awards and rewards throughout the season. These culminate in the end-of-season awards, usually presented at the team banquet. But all season long, to keep the athletes motivated and positive, awards and rewards are effective. As any coach, teacher, or parent knows, positive reinforcement, done the right way, works!

Beginning with the first week of coach-led practice in the summer, institute an Athlete of the Week award(s). If funds are available, purchase special t-shirts with Athlete of the Week printed on the front or back with the school logo. Be mindful of issuing these to a variety of your runners. The top runners always work hard and do as directed. It does not mean they cannot receive an award occasionally. However, top runners are going to get lots of honors and attention during the racing season. It is the mid-range and back-of-the-pack runners who need acknowledgment for their hard work, progress, work through injury, personal records (PRs), and great attitudes.

Secret Sisters is a popular team-bonding idea that many female runners love. The captains, with the coach's guidance, organized and ran this tradition. Secret Sisters involved some random way of assigning each runner another team member to be her "secret sister." The pairings are kept confidential until the end of the season banquet. Only captains need to know who has who so they can monitor the giving. At each meet for the season, athletes bring a small anonymous "gift" to be passed out by the captains prior to the first race. Emphasize that the gift should not be costly. Specify what that means and provide examples like: sports drinks with a special note or a favorite energy bar with an inspirational quote. The captains must monitor the participants to make sure they remember to bring the gifts. Captains should have some spare gifts in case someone forgets. My teams brought a special thank you gift to the banquet when the secret sister identities were revealed.

As discussed earlier Speeding Tickets were awarded after each race. This was used to reward those runners making big improvements and who often came from further back in the pack. The entire team cheered when those athletes were recognized.

The Anchor Award highlighted fifth runners who made a difference for their team in a given race.

As part of the season-end banquet (more to come in a moment), the coaches gave out six to eight plaques to top athletes. We did not have set criteria for those awards. Each year, we would flex according to each unique group of athletes. Here is the basic list of award categories:

- Most Valuable Runner
- Newcomer of the Year (one or two awarded)

- Most Improved (could be within a year or from season to season)
- Most Inspirational
- Coaches' Award (a catch-all used for a variety of characteristics or performances)

Varsity Letters

There are as many ways of awarding these special letters as there are programs and coaches. Decide what you think best fits your philosophy and your program. Make sure it remains special. Some coaches have no particular criteria. Other programs make letters based on a complicated point system for participation, races run, points scored, and honors won. Some establish a minimum time standard that must be met, regardless of races in which a runner has participated. Have your criteria clearly documented and distributed at the start of the season to minimize complaints. (See **Appendix 9** for a sample.)

I basically gave letters to eight to ten runners a year out of a team of fifty to eighty members. My criteria: They had to have run in at least one varsity race or have been eligible to run in a varsity race but were asked to stay at a lower level to ensure a team win. More than one varsity race run would automatically result in a letter. There was no time standard.

Senior Letters

When we began to be successful and have numerous top runners in the CVHS program, a non-varsity upperclassman raised the issue of the extreme difficulty found in earning a varsity letter in our program, and many excellent runners were missing out. If a runner had been at another, less accomplished program, she would have been a varsity runner. Eventually, a varsity letter was awarded to those who had been with the CVHS program for four years and had participated in 80 percent of races. This was known as the "Senior Letter" because of how it was earned, although it was the same varsity letter.

CHAPTER 17:

THE BANQUET

Celebrating the Season

There is a saying among coaches: The season is not over until the banquet is over.

The banquet certainly evolved over the course of my thirty-plus years of coaching. Early on, my wife Melisa would do the cooking, serving, decorating, and then help pass out the awards. She asked the custodial staff to set up tables and chairs in our school's multipurpose area. By the end of my career, the wonderful Booster Club parents held the banquet at a country club or hotel with catered food in a professionally-decorated room. The parents handled all the arrangements: reserving the site, sending the invitations, and setting up/cleaning up. It was always a beautiful event. As my career progressed, I had an enjoyably small part to play in the banquet due to the parents' efforts. I was able to focus on celebrating the athletes rather than being an event planner.

I will assume for the purposes of this writing that you are starting out as a banquet organizer. Here are some things to consider as you prepare your season-end celebration. (Keep in mind: I specifically coached the girls' team only, but our banquet combined both the boys' and girls' teams.)

Site

Depending on money and the size of team, the options range from an on-campus event to hosting it a restaurant, hotel, or club. Plan ahead by reserving the location three to six months ahead of time.

Food

Money and numbers often dictate the food, too. It can be catered, potluck, or dessert only. Perhaps the Boosters will offset the ticket price. There should be accommodations for those unable to pay.

Date

It is ideal to have the Banquet date and location in place at the start of the season, printed on the schedule, and available on the website. The CVHS Banquet was always the week after the State Meet, in early December.

Participants and Invites

All athletes and families should be invited. If it's a potluck, you will need to figure out how much of various kinds of foods should be available. If food is to be provided by a paid service, you will need paid reservations weeks in advance. Begin early with the invitations and commitments. Outside vendors will likely need a deposit of some sort. The CVHS Boosters paid for all athletes and coaches and only charged other family members. Even if there is no Booster Club, enlist the help of a parent-led committee.

Varsity Letters, Certificates of Participation, Scholar Athletes, and Awards

At CVHS, one month before the Banquet, the athletic director asked me who would receive Varsity Letters and Certificates of Participation. CUSD also provided a scholar Athlete Award based on grade point averages for varsity athletes. The Coach Plaques, discussed previously, were created by an outside vendor. Make a list and set some dates to get these things done on time.

Photo Albums

The CVHS parents made special photo albums. It was labor intensive but very meaningful. Parents would volunteer by gender and level or grade to take pictures at all the meets, some practices, and pre-meet dinners. They would then meet prior to the banquet and put together a bound photo album for *every* individual athlete on the team with pictures featuring them. These albums were gifted to the athletes as they arrived at the banquet.

The Agenda and the Program

Decide with your assistant coaches, parents, and athletes, what you want to emphasize at the banquet and in the program. Who should be honored? How much time do you want to take up? Often, these banquets take place on a school night, so be sensitive to finishing at a reasonable hour. I have heard of athletic banquets taking four to five hours, which I think is too long.

Here is the CVHS general Banquet Agenda:
- 6:00 Welcome by Head Coach and Booster President
- 6:15 Begin Dinner Service
- 7:00 Begin Program
- 7:00 Introductions: Coaches and Boosters

- 7:05 Booster Presidents: Thank yous for key parents that worked on meets, dinners, photos, and gifts to coaches from parents
- 7:20 Coaches Presentations: alternating male and female teams
  - Scholar Athletes
  - Captains
  - Seniors
  - All League and County recognition
  - Certificates of Participation for non-varsity—by level: Frosh, Soph, Junior Varsity, Senior Letters, Varsity Letters, and CIF and State certificates
  - Special Plaque Awards
- 8:30 Athlete's Presentation to Coaches
- 8:45 Closing

CHAPTER 18:

POST SEASON AND TRANSITION TO TRACK AND FIELD

The CVHS program in post-season was governed under the rules of our school, district, and CIF section. Your situation may vary depending on your school rules and your personal philosophy.

It is especially important that the runners take a break both physically and mentally after the season. A consensus of coaches and studies based on research would suggest a two-to-three-week break. This could involve complete rest for the entire time with a gradual reintroduction of running two or three times a week for another two weeks. To be honest, it also gives the coach(es) some time away from the sport and the athletes, which can be refreshing for everyone.

My teams had the added element of a report card grade to consider. The student-athletes were still in class when the season was over—with a month left to go until the semester ended. Our school site and the athletic director allowed the runners to rest for two weeks.

They met only on the designated attendance days, three times a week due to our block scheduling. The runners sat and did homework.

In the post-season, I had the wonderful opportunity to coach ten to twelve runners who were competing for several more weeks with the hopes of making it to the State Meet. The remainder of the team (forty to sixty girls) were not required to meet. That meant that for three weeks (including Thanksgiving week), the non-racing girls were off while the racing athletes were in training. After Thanksgiving and the State Meet until end of semester (prior to winter break) the CIF/State athletes were on rest. The non-CIF/State athletes returned to maintenance running three times a week.

During this post-season period, I needed to determine which runners I would invite to join the distance team for track and field in the spring. Given our large numbers (fifty to eight) at cross country, it was not practical to have all runners participate in distance at track and field. There are several reasons for this.

First, there is only so much space on the track for athletes to practice. Sprinters and hurdlers need to be working in lanes on the track almost daily. At CVHS, this would be an average of fifty athletes. This limits the availability of lanes for distance runners to use on a daily basis. The second reason is that given the nature of scoring at track and field meets, less athletes are needed in any specific event. In dual meets, only three places score from both teams combined. In larger invitational meets, only eight to ten athletes can score in any individual race. Freshman would sometimes want to try out for other events at track and field. Sprinting is often attractive; some may wish to try the jumps or the hurdles, and others see themselves as pole vaulters.

CHAPTER 19:

DISTANCE TEAM AT TRACK AND FIELD

Once you know your distance team members, communicate a transition training schedule to them. As explained in the previous chapter, there are different philosophies for how to proceed during this period, as well as considerations regarding your area's or state's schedule. Some coaches prefer a week of complete rest and then a resumption of running several days a week. Other coaches advocate for two weeks of complete rest, a week of minimal running, and then a slow weekly buildup of mileage toward the spring track and field season.

Much of the country has an indoor season between cross country and track and field, the West, California in particular, does not have such a season. Whatever your particular yearly schedule may be like, runners need some rest and recovery time between seasons. I will share the approach I took based on the schedule that we followed in California.

We began our training in July, culminating with our State Championship on Thanksgiving weekend. Our track and field training formally began when second semester started in early January—after the holiday vacation. Since the distance team for track and field was dominated by runners who had likely trained and raced well into November, I gave them two weeks off from running. This took them into mid-December. Then during their vacation, I would suggest a plan with three to four runs a week, all at an easy pace—two runs of thirty to forty minutes and two at forty to fifty minutes. Once they returned to school in early January, they would have had about three weeks rebuilding their base.

The distance team at track and field generally runs the 800-, 1600-, and 3200-meter events. Some states have relay events, including the 4x800 and the distance medley relay (1200, 400, 800, and 1600) as part of their regular schedule of events. In California, those events were featured in invitationals but not in CIF and state competitions. When considering the training schedule for the distance team, the coach has to consider that training for the 800 and 3200 are substantially different. The 800 requires more frequent and shorter speed workouts on top of an endurance base, where the 3200 is more like cross country training with more emphasis on long runs and tempo runs—especially early in the season—and then track-specific speed work later in the training cycle.

Coaches have to decide how to approach training for these three different events, and there are several considerations that impact the chosen approach. Are runners going to be mainly doing single events in meets, or will they be doubling or even tripling? Sometimes, that is a function of the size of the team, as well. Smaller distance teams may need runners to be in multiple distance events. This would necessitate a training approach that prepared them for at least two, if not all three, of the distances mentioned above. If, on the other hand, runners are more likely to be doing just one event, their training could focus mainly on that one event.

Once you have assessed your team size and decided on the approach you will take toward singling or athletes running multiple events in races, then you can establish the overall approach to training you will take. If you are going to have runners doing multiple events over a season—and especially if they may be doing all three race distances over the course of a season—your approach should be to train them for all three events. This can be done in two ways.

First, train everyone like a 1600-meter runner. This will provide a balance between the strength and endurance of the 3200-meter runner and the speed of the 800-meter runner. A second approach is to have a two-week training cycle where workouts specific to each distance event are performed in a rotating fashion. For example, assuming twelve workouts in a two-week span, four would be shorter, more intense speed workouts for an 800-meter runner. Four workouts would be longer distance and tempo runs for the 3200-meter runner, and the remaining four workouts would be for the combination of strength and speed a 1600-meter runner needs.

Who should run which events? Assessing talent and placing them in the correct events is a challenge. Most of the time, runners will fall into two groups. These will be your groups if you separate your runners by events for training purposes. More on this in a moment. The two groups would be 800/1600-meter runners and 1600/3200-meter runners. Obviously in the case of returning runners you know what they can do and where they likely belong. For freshman or newcomers, you can use the athletes results from races and workouts during the cross-country season to help determine their correct event group placement for the distance team at track and field. Athletes who seemed to perform significantly better in workouts at shorter intervals, like the 200, 300, or 400 meters, than at longer ones are likely your

800/1600 runners. Conversely, runners whose long runs and tempo runs seem better than their shorter intervals are your 1600/3200 runners. Also recalling the runner's general placement during the flying 40s and 60s proscribed in the training sections of the book can be another indicator of their natural proclivities.

Make no mistake, most runners are better suited to one of those groupings than the other. Haley Herberg, our 2017 California State cross country champion and now runner at University of Washington, is a classic example of this. With a high school personal best of 16:01 for three miles, 10:08 for 3200 meters, and 4:47 for 1600 meters, various charts would predict her 800-meter time to be at or below 2:15. Though she did not compete in the event, often her best was around 2:18. Her strength was her strength, not her short speed.

CASE STUDY: NATALIE HERBERG
Speed to Burn!

Natalie started her running career at Capistrano Valley with an established record as an age-group competitor in the South Orange County area. She had a steady progression from a solid 19:31 best as a freshman to 18:51 as a sophomore and on to 18:01 as a junior. She had a spectacular senior year where she broke a longstanding meet record and ended up with a personal record of 17:19.

As outstanding as her cross-country career was, however, it was her work on the track that brought her a scholarship to run for the California Bears cross country and track and field teams. Natalie was a tall, powerful runner with a lot of natural speed. As described in Chapter 17, her short interval work at cross country and astonishing kick to finish races clearly identified her as an 800/1600 runner at track and field. Because of her work at cross country, she had tremendous endurance, which translated into the ability to do some high volume and high-quality workouts during the track season. Natalie became an 800-meter specialist, and during her junior year, I trained her specifically for that race. I used a combination of workouts from 400-meter workouts of short, intense speed to 1600-meter workouts for endurance and pace. She would also anchor our 4x400 team, running splits in the fifty-eight second range.

Natalie eventually broke the school record for 800 meters, which still stands at 2:11.92 and qualified for the California State Meet finals as a junior.

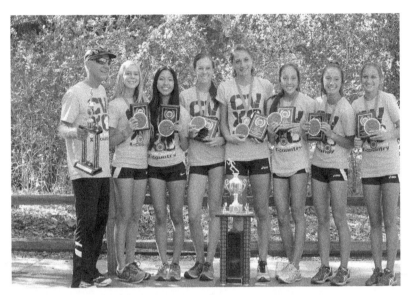

OCC 2013, Natalie is in the middle

Just as I did with the cross-country season calendar, I counted backward from the culminating races that I wanted to have the runners peaked for. A significant difference here between cross country and track and field is that you may have top individuals whose season may be three or four weeks longer than their teammates as they advance into post-season competition. Because I had the good fortune of often having CIF Southern Section finalists and even State Meet qualifiers as individuals, I would have to plan their training cycles somewhat differently than the remainder of the team, who would likely finish their seasons at the league finals. However, I did this adjustment about halfway through the training cycle so that all the athletes would be doing roughly the same training schedule before those adjustments were necessary. In California, our State Meet was in early June, preceded by a section state-qualifying meet, a section championship week, and a section preliminary week. That is four weeks of training following our league finals. Beginning in late December, there would be about twenty weeks of training through the league finals.

Because the main focus of this book is on cross-country, I am going to give just a brief overview of the training calendar for the distance team at track and field. Just like with cross country, think of the season as having several phases that focus on different workouts to develop different energy systems and race skills.

The first, lasting seven to eight weeks, is the Base Phase. This will be much like the early summer in cross country with distance runs and long runs becoming the key workouts. This would be followed by the Strength Phase, not unlike the second phase of cross country with tempo runs as a key workout but with longer speed intervals(800s) being introduced earlier here than in cross country. This phase would be five to six weeks long, depending on your overall schedule. If you were going to separate into two training groups (800/1600 and 1600/3200), this would be where you would begin to do this.

Next would be seven to eight weeks of developing speed. This is where you would be beginning early-season practice meets and invitationals. The focus here would turn away from the longer runs and more to several sessions a week of shorter intervals (200s and 400s), depending on the 8/16 or 16/32 groupings. Finally, you finish with a three-week peaking phase, which often coincides for the elite runners with their post-league sectional and state competitions. This phase has high intensity and low volume workouts with distance runs, even for 3200-meter runners substantially reduced.

Here is a sample week from the middle of Phase 1, The Base Phase

- Monday: 45-minute run
- Tuesday: 7-minute speed ladder (see Chapter 2)
- Wednesday: 45-minute run
- Thursday: Hill repeats (see Chapter 2)

- Friday: Cross train, pool work, or 30-minute run
- Saturday: Long run for 55–60 minutes

Here is a sample from the middle of Phase 2, The Strength Phase

- Monday: 8x1000 at Tempo Pace (see Chapter 8)
- Tuesday: 40–45-minute recovery run
- Wednesday: 7x150 all-out with walking between
- Thursday: 40–45-minute recovery run
- Friday: 6x300 at 800 paces
- Saturday: Long run for 65–75 minutes

Here is a sample from the middle of Phase 3, The Speed Development Phase

- Monday: 9x300 at 800 paces
- Tuesday: 40–45-minute recovery run
- Wednesday: 6x800 at 3200 pace or 12x400 at 1600 pace
- Thursday: 35–40-minute recovery run
- Friday: Pre-meet
- Saturday: Invitational races

Here is a sample from the middle of Phase 4, The Peaking Phase

- Monday: 40–45-minute recovery run (assuming Saturday race)
- Tuesday: 6x400 at near 800 paces
- Wednesday: 30–35-minute recovery run and 6 flying 40's
- Thursday: 6x150 all-out or 2x800 between 1600 and 3200 paces
- Friday: Pre-meet
- Saturday: Post-season competition

For more details and complete workouts for the Track and Field season, see my website, www.coachrunwin.com.

CHAPTER 20:

DESIGNING COURSES AND MANAGING RACES

How to Organize Chaos

O ver my thirty-four years of coaching cross country, I have had to design, set up, and mark courses nearly one hundred times. These have ranged from dual meet and league finals courses on campuses and in parks to community 5k race courses. I have served as the meet manager or race director for many of these races. What follows in this chapter is the basic outline of how to design courses and manage races on them.

Make sure that whether you are a coach, parent, athlete, or volunteer, you check with your school, league, region, and state for any rules regarding course setup and management of races. A good resource is the *NFHS Rule Book for Track and Field and Cross Country,* which has a section specifically on course set-up and management.

Course Design and Set-Up

You need to decide what type of course you want to create. Do you want it to be flat and fast or challenging? Once you have made that basic choice, then you can focus on surfaces and measurement as you will see. It is also important to assess the area to be used to determine if the course will be an out-and-back course or some form of a loop.

An important consideration in course creation and race management is safety. Surfaces, even if challenging due to elevation changes, slopes, and thick grass or dirt, need to be safe for runners. They should be void of rocks and gravel—unless very tiny and unlikely to cause twisted ankles or substantial injury with a fall.

Most courses, whether by planned design or necessity of the site, use a variety of surfaces. This can be a positive factor in creating unique racing circumstances.

The course should be coach- and spectator-friendly. For safety reasons, runners should not be placed in situations where they cannot be reached quickly in case of an emergency. Courses should be user friendly for coaches and spectators to move from place to place, safely and easily. Coaches can communicate and monitor runners' progress and spectators can cheer more often when the course has been set up to allow movement from place to place.

In most of the world, cross country courses are on mainly dirt and grassy surfaces. These are more forgiving on runners' bodies than harder surfaces. Weather is more likely to negatively impact these softer surfaces, however. But for many runners, coaches and spectators of cross country, the impact of weather on the surfaces and during the race is part of the challenge and even the fun of the sport.

If hard surfaces, like concrete or asphalt, have to be used, try to minimize the amount of those surfaces. Studies have shown that concrete has the worst impact on runners' bodies so asphalt is a better choice, if you're given one. If actual asphalt or concrete highways have to be used, be conscious of the canter or slant of most roads designed to help with rain runoff into gutters. Extensive running on a slant can lead to injury fairly quickly as the runners are imbalanced and overstressing one side versus the other.

When measuring the course, use a calibrated wheel, if possible. They can be purchased from most track and cross-country equipment suppliers. I have used my GPS watch at times. I once set up a 5k community course and used the calibrated wheel and GPS at same time. My watch was as accurate as the wheel, but make sure that your watch is, in fact, accurate before relying on it if accuracy is a prime concern. If you are setting up a course where records need to be certi-fied to be official, you will need to pay a professional to measure and certify the distance.

Setting up the start and finish areas is important for safety as well as for facilitating the fairest competition. The start area should be wide enough to allow all teams two or three competitors at the start line. Ideally, a full varsity team of seven can all be on the starting line together. If each runner needs two to three feet to freely operate, as-sess how many teams or runners will be on the line in any given race and create a start area wide enough to facilitate them. The start area should not narrow down for at least one hundred meters— preferably 150 to 200 meters—to allow plenty of time for runners to spread out and avoid tripping and falling, which would necessitate a race restart.

The finish area should have a straightaway of at least 150 meters out from the finish line itself. The finish chute should begin about twenty-five feet from the finish line with flags or ropes on both sides to keep spectators away from runners. The finish chute should narrow from fifteen feet wide at the finish line to three feet wide by the end of the one hundred feet so that competitors can be lined up correctly in order of finish before they depart the finish chute.

When designing the course, try to make sure turns are wide and continuous. Avoid U-turns whenever possible as they slow down the runners. If they are necessary, try to make them as long as possible and not an abrupt about-face.

There are formal rules about marking a race course. See the above referenced NFHS rule book. In general, try to have flags, cones, and signs that can be seen from at least one hundred feet away. In setting up and marking courses over the years, I have used colored flags, cones of all sizes, and tape on hard surfaces. Many people use chalk on hard surfaces. Make sure that your use of chalk is permitted and that it can be easily cleaned up when your race is finished. Mile markers can be handmade, actual timing clocks, or purchased from track and cross-country equipment suppliers. Directional signs can be made or purchased in similar ways.

I followed some basic common-sense guidelines in marking the courses. You want runners to be absolutely clear about where they can and cannot run. Runners should not have to hesitate or think about where they are going, even if it is the first time they are running the course. It makes the runners happier, results in faster times, and avoids a lot of conflict and grief that may come from runners going the wrong way on an unmarked or unclear course. I tried, when possible to follow the same procedures of cone and flag placement throughout a course. For example, if possible, I would have all of the cones or flags on the left so runners always knew to run to the right of those cones or flags. Sometimes, you can create a tunnel to direct runners with flags or cones on both sides. At turns, post directional signs, especially if it is an intersection used several times. (Try to avoid those.)

If your course is at your school or a local park, make sure athletes and spectators have access to bathrooms and water fountains. If you are using an undeveloped lot or will not have access to restrooms, you will need to order some portable bathrooms (porta-potties). Many companies will deliver and pickup for you. Cost can vary, but they are not expensive to use.

Race Management

Make sure you are clear about any permits or permissions you may need for your course and your race. If you are racing at your school site, make sure you are on the calendar. Have the AD or the activities director point you to the correct forms to fill out and file. If you are off campus at a local park or community center, make sure that you have contacted all possible authorities to ask for permission. These may include the city, parks and recreation, county trails and parks, the fire department, the police department, and even the health department. Some offsite permits may require insurance coverage from your school or school district. All off-campus paperwork should be done months ahead of time so plan ahead.

You will need to decide how you are going to have the race timed. There are basically two options: hand-timing with stop watches or electronic timing. Electronic timing can be with your own equipment or through a hired professional timing company.

If you are just doing a dual meet and/or have some challenges financially, the hand-timing route is for you. Have at least two watches running so you have a back-up. There are many high-quality stopwatches on the market. There are small watches that include recall features to get each individual finisher's time and larger ones that have a small printer included that prints out a tape of the results for each runner. One simple way to score using hand-timing is as follows:

- Give each finisher a stick or three-by-five card with a number on it, the numbers indicating their order of finish.
- Write the names and order of finish down on a spreadsheet

- Match the times from the stopwatches with the places in order of finish
- Score the meet as explained in an earlier chapter

With electronic or automatic timing, you can purchase your own system for as little as $500—one with basic timing and scoring capabilities. Having your own system that works for track meets as well and comes with cameras, scoreboards, etc., can cost as much as $20,000. Hiring a professional timing company just for a dual cross country meet or league meet may cost anywhere from $400 to $800, depending on where you live and the number of teams and runners. The basic package usually includes, timing and results, a finish clock, and perhaps a large display screen. Some companies have live apps so everyone can track results on their devices. You can also request, usually at an additional cost, mile clocks. Make sure you are clear about whether they provide the bibs or chips to record the runners' times and places. Most companies are now providing chips that are worn on the shoes and is part of the cost. Make sure that you provide adequate time and direction for teams to get their entries to you or to the timing company.

Having a certified trainer/first-aid person on site is usually required by school administrations or in the case of a community race, the local authorities. Make it clear to teams and spectators where that person or group is located (usually near finish line). This can be done with course and site maps and with signs on site. The trainer may come with ice and fluids but verify they do, especially in hot or humid weather.

Other equipment to consider are tables and chairs for the finish area and scoring area, a sound system to announce upcoming races and results, and walkie talkies to communicate around the course. It is also a good idea to have a tent at the finish line. Hired timers may have their own, but certainly if weather is an issue (hot or wet), you want to have the timers and scorers protected. Often teams have their own well marked tents, and it's nice advertising for the team as well as a clear identifier of where the start and/or finish line is located. Though everyone has a cell phone these days, remote sites for races may not have coverage, and thus, the walkie talkies can be a useful safety and communication tool.

Finally, as the saying goes, "It takes a village!" Even for a small dual meet, you need ten to twenty volunteers to help with timing, course marshalling, chute management, and course set-up and break-down. Your league or regional association may require you to have an official starter or referee. If so, they usually need to be booked well in advance. There should be a volunteer placed about 150 meters from the start whose job is to signal the starter to recall the race (usually by firing the starting gun again) if someone falls down in the starting area. This starter/referee can also serve as the finish line judge in case there are issues regarding the order of finish. At every crucial turn or intersection where runners could make a wrong turn—in addition to your signs, flags, and cones—you should have a course marshal to direct runners. Certainly, if there is an area where runners could be impacted by vehicle traffic, there should be a traffic marshal. Many teams and races will have volunteers from each team meet before-hand to discuss assignments and go over course maps. Make sure you have maps and assignments printed and ready to pass out at this meeting.

You will also need volunteers working the finish chute. You should have at least four for a small meet and as many as ten for a larger one. They should spread out along the chute, helping to keep runners in correct order of finish and assisting anyone who may need help as they move through the chute to the scorer's table.

When the meet has concluded, make sure you have a crew prepared to clean up the course and remove all markings, cones, flags, signs, and chalk so the facility is in the same condition—if not better—than when the meet began.

CHAPTER 21

VIRTUAL COACHING

When You Can't Be There in Person

This book was written during the year 2020 and finished in early 2021. I have specifically chosen not to incorporate COVID-19 references in the hope that the content will have a more universal and long-lasting appeal. However, one thing that will be an ongoing tool for coaches and runners in the future will be virtual coaching.

What I mean by virtual coaching is any and all coaching tools and methods designed to allow coaches and their runners to work together remotely, without being in physical proximity. There are many websites runners can use to look up workout plans for any race distance. My own website, www.coachrunwin.com has them. I am not referring to those when I talk about virtual coaching. I am referring more specifically to tools used to link coach and runner together in an online dialogue.

I am sure that Zoom became part of most people's lives as 2020 moved into 2021. The free app provides a video-chatting service that allows up to one hundred participants concurrently. I know most coaches I communicated with during 2020 were using Zoom to communicate with their athletes. There are other tools available, as well; here are several:

- WhatsApp: a Facebook-owned app available on the web or your smartphone. It allows you to send SMS messages for free and supports group chats of up to 256 people.
- Facebook Messenger: supports up to six people on screen during a video call
- FaceTime: Apple's take on video-conferencing, supporting up to thirty-two callers at once
- Google Duo: a simple, useful, but minimal video-calling app for up to twelve on one call

In addition to these platforms to facilitate the communication between coach and runner, there are some additional tools I would recommend, which extremely helpful in making the virtual coaching experience beneficial. Primary among these is VDOT O2, a custom training application for runners. It was created by the Run SMART Project and legendary coach Dr. Jack Daniels. Remember my discussion in Chapter 2 of how I used his running research and formulas for my own training system? VDOT O2 helps runners determine their proper training paces, logs that data, and provides instant feedback. See their website for complete information on the program and how to use it.

As a coach, you can sign up and pay a monthly fee (around $20) to use the service with and for your runners. It does not cost the runners anything. You email them information to log in, and when they do, they answer a couple of basic questions. Then you're ready to have a virtual coaching relationship. It does require them to have some sort of smartwatch or phone that can upload their data after each workout.

It supports Garmin Connect and Strava devices. It takes just minutes to have coaches and athletes up and running! VDOT 02 tracks weekly mileage. It allows the coach to customize workouts for each individual or for the entire team in just a few minutes. Coaches can give immediate feedback about completed workouts. Training paces for athletes are updated based on recent workout and race results. This is an automatic feature based on Dr. Daniels's forty years of research. **Table 1** is the simple one-page reference, adapted from Dr. Daniels's work for determining workout paces as I explained in Chapter 2. I have a colleague and friend, Bob Price of San Juan Hills High School, who used the VDOT 02 system with his athletes during the summer of 2020 to keep them on task during uncertain times.

Here are some additional apps that can be used by individuals:

- Couch to 5k: many unique features, like training plans designed by Active.com. You can hear human audio cues that guide you through workouts and calculate your distance and pace and map routes with free GPS support.
- Nike Run Club: a running app for iPhone and Apple Watch that has GPS tracking details and customized coaching plans to fit your goals and adapt to your progress.

Google Docs and Microsoft Word Online have helpful tools for sharing data between runners and coaches. A coach can send out a template with workout goals. The runners then fill in their times and distances when workouts are completed. Runners can make comments about their workouts, and coaches can respond on the same document. These are excellent and useful tools that are not just one format or formula. They can be adapted to the specific approaches and needs of individual coaches and their runners.

RESOURCES

You can find these downloadable resources on my website, www. coachrunwin.com. Further resources are listed in the Appendices that follow.

- A Sample Workout Goal Sheet
- Pre- and Post-Workout Routines
- Pace, Distance, and Time Chart
- Sample Season Summary of Times
- Sample State Meet Goals' Sheet
- Pre-Summer Workouts
- A Summer Workout Plan
- Summer Miles Run Sample
- Mammoth Camp Selection Grid

CAPO VALLEY LADY COUGAR CROSS COUNTRY TRAINING SYSTEM

Overall Philosophy

Each individual athlete is provided with the appropriate paces, distances, numbers of repeats, or intervals, based on their own stage of development, which data collection indicates at any one moment of time and usually adjusted weekly. The basic unit of comparison is time of work effort in a workout.

Example: An athlete doing 5x 1000 tempo intervals in five minutes each is doing twenty-five minutes of individual appropriate work. This is basically *equal* to an athlete doing 4x6 minutes or 7x3:30 minutes.

To have athletes of varying physical abilities and development do the same exact paces and same number of intervals or repeats is detrimental to *everyone*—could be too slow for top or way too fast or too long for slower runners.

1. Pyramid of training phases

a. Four phases of training in a season. Each has different emphasis with certain workouts taking prominence over others in each phase.

   1. Base Phase: emphasis on long runs and mileage build-up—8 weeks

      a. Purpose is to build more mitochondria cells that transport oxygen and blood to muscles. More miles and long runs build more of this energy transport system

   2. Strength Phase: tempo and hill work with beginnings of some speed development—6 weeks, long run becomes secondary

      a. Purpose is to increase the anaerobic or lactate threshold, the speed and effort at which you are just on the edge of being out of breath. This is the most crucial workout for the three-mile/5k distance but is built on top of long runs and miles

   3. Speed Work: race-pace speed work, like repeat 800s or 400s—five weeks, no long run, just medium recovery run

      a. Purpose is to increase ability to sustain race pace speed

   4. Peaking and Tapering: decrease in mileage, increase or maintenance of intensity—two or three weeks

      a. a. purpose is to maximize ability to race and recover during championship season

b. Types of workouts in general with associated paces and percentage of VO2 Max heart rate

1. Long runs and recovery runs: talking or aerobic paces, 1:30 to 2 min over three-mile race pace, 65–75 percent of max

2. Tempo runs: typically 1000s at 82–87 percent of max, about 24–30 seconds slower than three-mile race pace. Tempo 1000s is done with short rests of 1–1:30 to prevent full recovery

3. Speed Development: flying 40's and speed ladder, trains form/muscles for running and racing under race pace without taxing aerobic system. Done at 92–100 percent of max at 400–1600-meter race paces.

4. Traditional Race Pace Repeats of Intervals: i.e., 6x800, 10x400, done at three-mile race or just under pace with equal to more rest to allow near full or full recovery.

c. Weekly and monthly training emphasis in miles and percentages

1. In Base Phase, virtually one hundred percent is at aerobic pace

2. In Strength Phase, 80–85 percent of miles is aerobic, 8–10 percent is tempo, 2–3 percent is speed development, i.e., for 35-mile-a-week runner, 28–30 is aerobic, 1–2 is speed development and 2–4 is tempo.

3. In Speed Phase, speed is 10–15 percent, speed development 2–3 percent, tempo 2–3 percent, aerobic 70–75 percent.

4. In Peaking and Tapering: 65–70 percent aerobic, 15–20 percent speed, 4–6 percent speed development.

2. **Designing individual workout plans so all can develop to the best of their individual capabilities**
   a. Collect data on each athlete from early summer distance and long runs, find average per mile pace.
   b. Using VDOT chart (adapted from Dr. Jack Daniels, *Running Formula*), assign VDOT number to athlete.
   c. Use the VDOT number to give range of pace for each workout.
   d. Record details of workouts for each athlete to monitor and adjust assigned VDOT and paces.
   e. Everyone does the workout that maximizes their individual development and success

APPENDIX 2

SAMPLE LADDER CHART

	Athlete	Grade	vdot	Dist	Pace		Pace Chart	
							Dist.	Pace
1		10	49	1.13	6:10			
2		11	40	.97	7:10		1.36	5:09
3		10	50	1.2	5:50		1.33	5:16
4		9	38	1.07	6:30		1.3	5:23
5		11	inj	inj	inj		1.27	5:30
6		10	35				1:23	5:40
7		10	39	.9	7:45		1.2	5:50
8		12	61	1.29	5:25		1.15	6:00
9		11	44	1.08	6:28		1.13	6:10
10		12	50	inj	inj		1.1	6:20
11		10	44	.98	7:05		1.07	6:30
12		9	35	.87	8:00		1.05	6:40
13		12	28	.5	14:00		1.02	6:50
14		9	39	.96	7:15		1	7:00

15		11	55	inj	inj		.97	7:10
16		12	50	inj	inj		.95	7:20
17		9	39	.97	7:10		.93	7:30
18		10	39				.91	7:40
19		11	38	1.05	6:40		.89	7:50
20		10	35				.87	8:00
21		11	42	1.13	6:10		.85	8:10
22		9	39	1.09	6:25		.84	8:20
23		9	42	1.06	6:35		.82	8:30
24			38	.94	7:25		.8	8:40
25		12	35	.97	7:10		.79	8:50
26		12	55	1.2	5:50		.77	9:00
27		10		.97	7:10		.76	9:10
28		10	35				.75	9:20
29		10	46				.73	9:30
30		10	52	1.2	5:50		.72	9:40
31		11	42	inj	inj		.71	9:50
32		12	41	1.05	6:40		.7	10:00
33		10	41	inj	inj			

CVHS CROSS COUNTRY
Practice Etiquette and Safety

Prepared by CVHS Boys' Coach Matt Soto

U nlike most sports, the majority of our practices involve being off campus. There are some inherent risks associated with this. Common sense and good safety practices are the easiest way to minimize the chance of anything going wrong. Understanding how to stay safe as well as being responsible and using your own good judgment on a daily basis will allow you to avoid any adverse situations.

ACT APPRORIATELY

Be aware of everything you say and do when we are out in our community. You are representing not only our program but the school as a whole, especially if you or someone you are with is wearing a school-related shirt. Even if you think no one is paying attention, people may still hear or see what you are doing.

BE COURTEOUS

We often share roads and trails with other bikers, walkers, runners, and even horses. Give enough room for them to pass by safely, run in a single file line to allow for more space, if necessary. Don't block paths or take up space unnecessarily when waiting at a stoplight or along a trail. If a horse is approaching in the opposite direction, *stop* where you are and wait for the okay from the rider that it is safe to continue. You are risking their safety by not yielding.

DON'T ENGAGE (with anyone attempting to taunt or provoke you)

Although rare, it may be possible that you encounter someone from another school or from within a passing car making comments or trying to get a response out of you as a runner—i.e., "Run Forest, run" or something similar. Do not attempt to respond or interact with them.

ALWAYS RUN ON THE SOFTEST SURFACE

Dirt is always the best surface to run on; it allows for the lowest impact to your body. Avoid concrete when possible. If multiple surfaces are available, choose the softest.

RUN WITH SOMEONE

Running with someone ensures you can alert each other to potential risks as they happen. Additionally, someone else will be aware of the situation in the event that you may require assistance.

FACE ONCOMING TRAFFIC

Always be on the side of the street where you can see cars coming toward you. Avoid situations where cars are coming from behind you, even on sidewalks. If there is no sidewalk, maintain at least two feet of distance from the side of the road.

BE AWARE OF BLIND CORNERS

Look out for bikers and other trail users around corners that you may not be able to see past. If you are in an area where there are cars, don't go into a blind turn toward incoming traffic. This is the exception to otherwise facing oncoming traffic.

DON'T ASSUME CARS KNOW WHAT YOU WILL DO

Keep in mind that drivers may not see you or be alert to your presence. Not all cars yield at crosswalks or turns like they should.

DON'T TRY TO BEAT TRAFFIC LIGHTS

Approach traffic lights with caution. Obey the walk/do not walk signals. Do not try to sprint across a light to beat it as it changes.

FOLLOW ALL TRAFFIC LAWS

Do not jaywalk, run into, or cut across streets. Act in accordance with all signs, such as in construction areas. Share sidewalks with other users.

DON'T USE HEADPHONES

Headphones limit your ability to be alert to your surroundings.

DON'T APPROACH WILDLIFE

Some trails around our area are also inhabited by coyotes, deer, and rattlesnakes. While encounters are not typical, respect their space, and do not attempt to interact with any wildlife.

DON'T CROSS RUNNING WATER

After periods of heavy rain, some trails surrounding our campus are subject to flooding, and streams may also appear. Do not attempt to cross rushing water, especially if it is deep enough that you cannot see the bottom.

BE ALERT TO CHANGING TRAIL CONDITIONS

Watch out for ruts, holes, low branches, puddles, or other obstructions along trails. Be careful in areas where there is unstable footing, such as rocky or sandy sections. Alert those around you of upcoming obstacles.

UNDERSTAND WHERE YOU ARE GOING

If you are unclear of the route, ask for clarification beforehand, or stay with someone who knows where they are going.

KNOW YOUR LIMITS

Do not overexert yourself unnecessarily. Be aware of weather conditions, such as extreme heat or humidity. Only go as far or as fast as you can safely do.

PRACTICE THE COUGAR WAY

Be cheerful and friendly, greet everyone you pass with a "good morning" or a "good afternoon."

APPENDIX 4

RACE DAY SCHEDULE FOR DANA INVITATIONAL

Saturday, Sep 22, 2018

8:45 a.m.: All athletes at CV site (come early to find us, we are usually at top of home stands)

9:00 a.m.: Secret Sisters

Senior Girls—Race is Division 2 at 10:15, leader Emma

- 9:15 To bathrooms
- 9:38 Begin 12-min warmup run on course
- 9:50 Drills, etc.
- 10:05 Racing ready and head to start area
- 10:10 Strides in start area
- **10:15 RACE**
- *Cheer junior girls! Then be ready to cheer the rest!*

Junior Girls—Race is Division 2 at 10:45, leaders Carly and Hailey K

- 9:45 To bathrooms
- 10:08 Begin 12-min warmup run on course
- 10:20 Drills, etc.
- 10:35 Racing ready and head to start area
- 1040 Strides in start
- **10:45 RACE**
- *Cheer sophomore girls! Then be ready to cheer the rest!*

Sophomore Girls—Race is Division 2 at 11:15, leaders Kami and Sophia

- 10:15 To bathrooms
- 10:38 12-min warmup
- 10:50 Drills, etc.
- 11:05 Race ready and head to start area
- 11:10 Strides in start
- **11:15 RACE**
- *Cheer frosh girls!*

Frosh Girls—Race is Division 2 at 11:45, leaders Midori and Baylee

- 10:45 To bathrooms
- 11:08 12-min warmup
- 11:20 Drills, etc.
- 11:35 Race ready and head to start area
- 11:40 Strides in start
- **11:45 RACE**

12:30 All team stretch-down and celebration, 12:45 "Go Cougars" Athlete Departure

APPENDIX 5

SAMPLE RACE SPLIT SHEET

visit www.coachrunwin.com
for a downloadable version

VARSITY											
	athlete	grade	vdot	Mile1	pos	Mile2	2 mi	pos	Mile3	**3 mi**	**pos**	**Team Results**
1												
2												
3												
JV											
	athlete	grade	vdot	Mile1	pos	Mile2	2 mi	pos	Mile3	**3 mi**	**pos**	**Team Results**
1												
2												
3												

SOPH

	athlete	grade	vdot	Mile1	pos	Mile2	2 mi	pos	Mile3	3 mi	pos	Team Results
1												
2												
3												

FROSH

	athlete	grade	vdot	Mile1	pos	Mile2	2 mi	pos	Mile3	3 mi	pos	Team Results
1												
2												
3												

APPENDIX 6

Athlete:		Race:		Date:
Course:				
Goal Time:		Goal Pace Overall:		First Mile:
Goal Place:				
Describe your race plan:				
Results	Time:	Place:		
Three things I did well:				
1				
2				
3				
Three things I need to improve:				
1				
2				
3				

A SAMPLE WEIGHT WORKOUT FOR INDIVIDUAL RUNNERS

(By One of Our Athletes)

1. Machine flat bench, light weight 10 reps (will increase to 12–15 repetitions [reps], more reps and lighter weight = lean muscle, good cardio)
2. Machine lat pull, light weight 10 reps (will increase to 12–15 reps, more reps and lighter weight = lean muscle, good cardio)
3. Machine lat pull downs, light weight 10 reps (will increase to 12–15 reps, more reps and lighter weight = lean muscle, good cardio)
4. Dumbbell curls, light weight 10 reps (will increase to 12–15 reps, more reps and light weight = lean muscle, good cardio)

5. Dumbbell tri extensions, light weight 10 reps (will increase to 12–15 reps, more reps and lighter weight = lean muscle, good cardio)

6. Power cleans and military: pick up 10-pound bar from ground, clean and jerk to chest, then press above head. This is done in one continuous motion. Great exercise to build legs, arms, back, and shoulders. In football builds, great explosion off the line. Light weight 10 reps (will increase to 12–15 reps, more reps and lighter weight = lean muscle, good cardio)

7. Ten (10) medicine ball toss: Ashley and I stand about 5–6 feet from one another, play catch for 20 seconds, paying close attention to explosive chest passes. On each throw, bend legs into a squatting position and standing close to one another, chest pass the ball in one motion. So the arms, chest, and legs get a workout.

8. Arm swings, hold two weights and swing arms in running motion

9. Leg extensions

10. Leg curls

11. Leg press

Each circuit will be eleven (11) exercises, and an athlete will do three (3) circuits. They will be done at a good pace to hit the cardio aspect of this workout as well. After three (3) circuits of weight training, the athlete then does the following CORE WORKOUT:

1. 50 crunches and 50 bicycle crunches

2. 10 reps on declined bench of sit ups with a 2-pound ball

3. 10 reps on crunch machine

LADY COUGAR CROSS COUNTRY

Course Requirements and Grading System

Grading is based solely on participating in workouts and meets and is not based on ability or run times. However, "participating" means participating fully, with maximum effort each day in practice and racing in the meets. Though injuries and illness are a part of sports, those injured or ill can*not* expect to receive the same grade as those who participate fully. In cross country, if you are not racing, for whatever reason, you cannot earn an *A* for that race. If you do not practice, you can't earn an *A* for that day. Those with injuries/ not participating will be provided with opportunities to help that will grant the ability to achieve a *B+* grade for those practices or meets.

CUTTING A WORKOUT is CHEATING

The first time, you will receive a warning. If it happens twice, you lose a grade and cannot participate in next meet (with loss of points). The third time, you will be dismissed from the team.

- Practices
  - ⇒ 10 pts for practicing fully
  - ⇒ 8 pts for present but not practicing due to injury or illness **(after 3 days, doctor or on-site trainer must verify injury)**
  - ⇒ 4 pts for injured or ill more than 3 days with no doctors note
  - ⇒ 2 pts for present but not dressed out with no excuse
  - ⇒ 0 pts for not present **(regardless of the reason)**
- Meets
  - ⇒ 100% of the meet total for racing
    88% of the meet total for excused(injury/illness) non racing but helps keep score or otherwise work meet
  - ⇒ 80% of the meet total for not having enough miles in but helps keep times
    70% of the meet total for excused non racing but does not help
  - ⇒ 0% of the meet total for absence (regardless of the reason) *
    *Athletes with club soccer schedules can have one meet exempt from this with advance notice and agreement by coaches
    Note: Absence due to illness/conflict from one meet would not likely impact overall grade

GRADING SYSTEM DETAILS:

In Season Practices: 60 at 10 each max = **600**

Invitationals:

⇒ Laguna Hills, Woodbridge, Dana Inv, 50 each

⇒ Orange County, 75

⇒ Mt Sac, 75

⇒ **Total Invitationals = 300**

League Meets

⇒ Cluster #1, 200

⇒ Finals, 250

⇒ **League Meet Totals = 450**

Post-Season practices

⇒ First 5 at 5 = 25

⇒ Next 10 at 10 = 100

⇒ **Total = 125**

Goal Sheets: 7x20 pts each = **140**

Donation Form = 50

Banquet = 60

Final Exam

⇒ 100 for long run, 100

⇒ 100 for mile run, 100

⇒ Total = **200**

TOTAL SEMESTER POINTS = 1925

A = **1733**

B = **1540**

C = **1348**

D = **1155**

LADY COUGAR CROSS COUNTRY LETTERING POLICY

Minimum Requirements to letter in Cross Country:
1. Remain academically eligible throughout the season.
2. Have no unexcused absences from the meets.
3. Have no unexcused absences from practice.
4. Display good sportsmanship at all practices, meets and team functions.
5. Meet at least one of the Varsity standards below.

Varsity Standards:
1. Qualify for the "official "CIF "team of ten
2. Qualify for the CVHS CIF team (usually twelve or thirteen) and have a minimum of three races under 19:30 minutes
3. Race in a varsity race

"Senior Letter"

1. Complete four years of Cross Country that includes an "honest effort" to practice and compete at the individual's highest level and participation in at least 75 percent of the races. This includes regular participation in the summer practices

The Coaching staff, at their discretion, may letter or choose to not letter any athlete due to circumstances not accounted for in these minimum standards

SCHOLAR ATHLETES—a district and CIF controlled policy

VARSITY ATHLETES ONLY—not senior letter winners

Previous semester only at 3.75 and above (so incoming frosh do not get)

TABLE 1

Training Paces Based on VDOTS

vdot	3mi race	5k race	per mile	E pace Dist/Rec	F paces over 800 ra				R paces near1600 race pa		
					200	300	400	600	200	300	400
70	14:00	14:29	4:40	6:15-35	29	45	1:02	1:33	32	48	1:05
69	14:15	14:45	4:45	6:20-40	30	46	1:03	1:34	32	49	1:06
68	14:30	15:01	4:50	6:25-45	30	46	1:04	1:36	33	49	1:07
67	14:45	15:16	4:55	6:30-50	31	47	1:05	1:38	33	50	1:08
66	15:00	15:32	5:00	6:35-55	31	48	1:06	1:40	34	51	1:09
65	15:15	15:47	5:05	6:40-7:00	32	49	1:07	1:42	34	51	1:10
64	15:30	16:03	5:10	6:45-7:05	32	50	1:08	1:44	35	52	1:11
63	15:45	16:18	5:15	6:50-7:10	33	51	1:09	1:45	35	53	1:12
62	16:00	16:34	5:20	6:55-7:15	34	52	1:10	1:46	36	54	1:13
61	16:15	16:50	5:25	7:00-7:20	34	52	1:11	1:47	36	55	1:14
60	16:30	17:05	5:30	7:05-25	35	53	1:12	1:48	36	56	1:15
59	16:45	17:20	5:35	7:10-30	36	54	1:13	1:49	37	57	1:16
58	17:00	17:36	5:40	7:15-35	36	55	1:13	1:50	38	58	1:17
57	17:15	17:52	5:45	7:20-40	37	56	1:14	1:53	38	59	1:18
56	17:30	18:07	5:50	7:25-45	37	57	1:15	1:55	39	60	1:19
55	17:45	18:23	5:55	7:30-50	38	57	1:16	1:55	39	61	1:20
54	18:00	18:38	6:00	7:35-55	38	58	1:17	1:57	40	62	1:21
53	18:18	18:57	6:06	7:40-8:00	39	59	1:18	1:59	40	63	1:22
52	18:35	19:15	6:12	7:45-8:05	40	60	1:19	2:01	41	64	1:23
51	18:54	19:34	6:18	7:50-8:10	40	61	1:20	2:03	42	65	1:24
50	19:14	19:55	6:25	7:55-8:15	41	62	1:22	2:05	43	66	1:25
49	19:35	20:17	6:32	8:00-8:20	41	63	1:23	2:07	44	67	1:27
48	19:55	20:37	6:39	8:07-8:27	42	64	1:24	2:09	44	68	1:29
47	20:18	21:01	6:46	8:15-8:35	42	65	1:25	2:11	45	70	1:31
46	20:40	21:24	6:53	8:22-8:42	43	66	1:26	2:13	46	71	1:33
45	21:05	21:50	7:01	8:30-8:55	44	67	1:28	2:15	47	72	1:35
44	21:30	22:16	7:10	8:40-9:05	44	68	1:30	2:17	48	73	1:37
43	21:55	22:42	7:18	8:50-9:15	45	69	1:32	2:19	49	74	1:39
42	22:23	23:11	7:28	9:00-9:25	45	70	1:33	2:21	50	75	1:41
41	22:52	23:49	7:37	9:10-9:35	46	71	1:34	2:23	51	76	1:43
40	23:20	24:10	7:47	9:20-9:45	46	71	1:35	2:24	52	77	1:45
39	23:50	24:4	7:57	9:30-9:55	47	72	1:36	2:26	53	79	1:47
38	24:22:00	25:14	8:07	9:40-10:10	48	73	1:37	2:28	54	81	1:49

Data in Table 1 was adapted with permission from J. Daniels,
Daniels' Running Formula, 2nd ed. (Champaign, IL: Human Kinetics, 2005), 52–55.

		I paces or 3mile/5k race paces						Tempo paces					
600	800	400	600	800	1000	1200	1600	800	1000	1200	1600	2mi.	vdot
1:37	2:10	1:11	1:46	2:22	2:58	3:34	4:46	2:38	3:15	3:47	5:12	10:36	70
1:39	2:12	1:12	1:47	2:24	3:00	3:37	4:50	2:38	3:17	3:51	5:16	10:44	69
1:41	2:14	1:13	1:48	2:26	3:02	3:40	4:53	2:40	3:20	3:55	5:20	10:52	68
1:42	2:16	1:14	1:49	2:28	3:04	3:43	4:57	2:42	3:22	3:59	5:25	11:02	67
1:43	2:18	1:15	1:51	2:30	3:07	3:45	5:00	2:44	3:24	4:03	5:29	11:12	66
1:44	2:20	1:16	1:54	2:32	3:10	3:48	5:05	2:46	3:27	4:07	5:33	11:18	65
1:45	2:22	1:17	1:55	2:34	3:12	3:52	5:10	2:48	3:30	4:11	5:37	11:26	64
1:46	2:24	1:18	1:57	2:36	3:15	3:56	5:15	2:50	3:33	4:15	5:41	11:32	63
1:48	2:26	1:19	1:59	2:38	3:19	4:00	5:20	2:52	3:36	4:19	5:45	11:40	62
1:50	2:29	1:20	2:01	2:40	3:22	4:05	5:25	2:54	3:39	4:23	5:50	11:50	61
1:52	2:31	1:21	2:02	2:42	3:25	4:09	5:30	2:56	3:42	4:27	5:55	12:00	60
1:54	2:33	1:22	2:03	2:44	3:28	4:12	5:35	2:58	3:45	4:31	6:00	12:10	59
1:56	2:35	1:23	2:04	2:46	3:30	4:15	5:40	3:00	3:48	4:35	6:05	12:20	58
1:58	2:37	1:24	2:05	2:48	3:33	4:18	5:45	3:02	3:50	4:39	6:10	12:30	57
1:59	2:39	1:26	2:06	2:52	3:35	4:21	5:50	3:04	3:53	4:43	6:15	12:40	56
2:00	2:42	1:27	2:07	2:54	3:38	4:24	5:55	3:06	3:57	4:47	6:20	12:50	55
2:02	2:44	1:28	2:08	2:56	3:41	4:27	6:00	3:08	4:00	4:51	6:25	13:00	54
2:04	2:46	1:30	2:09	3:00	3:45	4:31	6:06	3:10	4:04	4:55	6:31	13:12	53
2:06	2:48	1:31	2:11	3:02	3:49	4:34	6:12	3:12	4:07	4:59	6:37	13:24	52
2:08	2:50	1:32	2:12	3:04	3:53	4:37	6:18	3:14	4:10	5:03	6:43	13:36	51
2:11	2:53	1:33	2:14	3:06	3:58	4:40	6:25	3:16	4:14	5:07	6:50	13:50	50
2:13	2:56	1:35	2:15	3:10	4:03	4:44	6:32	3:18	4:18	5:11	6:57	14:04	49
2:15	3:00	1:37	2:16	3:14	4:08	4:48	6:39	3:20	4:22	5:15	7:04	14:18	48
2:17	3:04	1:39	2:18	3:18	4:13	4:53	6:46	3:22	4:27	5:20	7:11	14:32	47
2:19	3:08	1:41	2:20	3:22	4:19	4:58	6:53	3:25	4:32	5:25	7:18	14:46	46
2:22	3:12	1:43	2:22	3:26	4:25	5:03	7:01	3:28	4:37	5:31	7:26	15:02	45
2:24	3:16	1:45	2:25	3:30	4:31	5:08	7:10	3:32	4:42	5:36	7:35	15:20	44
2:26	3:20	1:47	2:28	3:34	4:37	5:13	7:18	3:36	4:47	5:42	7:43	15:36	43
2:28	3:25	1:49	2:31	3:38	4:43	5:19	7:28	3:40	4:52	5:48	7:53	15:52	42
2:31	3:30	1:51	2:34	3:42	4:49	5:25	7:37	3:44	4:57	5:54	8:02	16:14	41
2:34	3:34	1:53	2:37	3:46	4:55	5:31	7:47	3:48	5:02	6:00	8:12	16:34	40
2:38	3:38	1:54	2:41	3:48	5:01	5:37	7:57	3:53	5:07	6:06	8:22	16:54	39
2:42	3:42	1:56	2:45	3:53	5:07	5:43	8:07	3:58	5:12	6:12	8:32	17:14	38

ABOUT THE AUTHOR

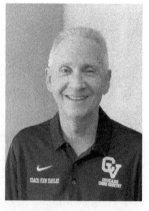

Ken Sayles spent over thirty years as the head girls' cross-country coach at Capistrano Valley High School (CVHS) in Mission Viejo, California. He was also the girls' track distance coach for twenty-seven years and served as the head girls' track and field coach for twenty-four years.

Following the 2014 season, in which his team was ranked as high as number eight in the nation, he was named Coach of the Year for Southern California by the California Coaches Association. CVHS competes in the most competitive area in the country, Southern California, and the most competitive subregion, Orange County, where he was named Coach of the Year by the *Orange County Register.*

Between 2012 and 2017, Capistrano Valley made the California State Meet six years in a row, a feat achieved by very few schools in California State Meet history. CVHS won the Orange County title twice and finished in the top three, six years in a row.

During his tenure, Coach Sayles coached one individual state cross-country champion and multiple Southern Section individual champions. In all, Coach Sayles coached over fifty individual South

Coast League and Orange County champions in cross country and track and field. In 2017, he had the unique distinction of having a female athlete qualify for Nike Cross Nationals (NXN) and a separate female athlete qualify for the Foot Locker Finals. In 2019, Coach Sayles helped a third female athlete compete at the Foot Locker Finals. As of this writing, he has four girls on Division 1 scholarships at universities in the Pac-12 conference, the toughest in the nation.

The first cross-country and track coach to be honored with the prestigious Southern Section of California's, Coaching with Character Award, Coach Sayles was commended because of the "Victory with Honor" emphasis he demonstrated in his coaching career. He also served as head of the Southern California Cross Country Coaches Association and was a member of the CIF Southern Section Cross Country Advisory Committee.

Mr. Sayles taught in the Social Science department at Capistrano Valley High for thirty-four years. He taught Advanced Placement (AP) Government and International Baccalaureate (IB) History of the Americas. He was twice named "Teacher of the Year" and went on to win the Capistrano Unified School District "Teacher of the Year" in 1999. He retired from the classroom in 2014 and stepped down as the full-time head coach in 2018. He now mentors a former star runner who is the new head coach.

"Coach" lives in Laguna Niguel California with his wife Melisa, a retired Spanish teacher and former assistant coach, and their Siberian husky, Luna. He serves as the volunteer race director for the BRAVE RACE 5k to benefit The Joyful Child Foundation—in memory of Samantha Runnion—which is a non-profit organization dedicated to the prevention of crimes against children.

A free ebook edition
is available with the
purchase of this book.

To claim your free ebook edition:
1. Visit MorganJamesBOGO.com
2. Sign your name CLEARLY in the space
3. Complete the form and submit a photo of the entire copyright page
4. You or your friend can download the ebook to your preferred device

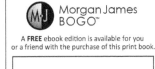

Morgan James BOGO™

A **FREE** ebook edition is available for you or a friend with the purchase of this print book.

CLEARLY SIGN YOUR NAME ABOVE

Instructions to claim your free ebook edition:
1. Visit MorganJamesBOGO.com
2. Sign your name CLEARLY in the space above
3. Complete the form and submit a photo of this entire page
4. You or your friend can download the ebook to your preferred device

Print & Digital Together Forever.

Snap a photo

Free ebook

Read anywhere

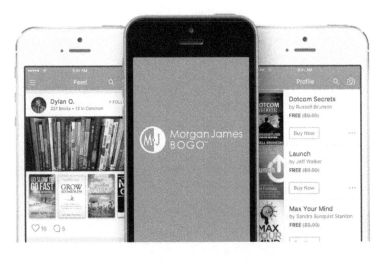